HOLISTIC DRUG & ALCOHOL REHABILITATION

Peter Lyndon-James

PO Box 1970, MIDLAND DC WA6936

Email orders: peter@lyndonjames.com.au

ISBN: 978-0-6453367-2-6

Scripture quotations marked (NIV) are taken from the Holy Bible, New International Version®, NIV®. Copyright © 1973, 1978, 1984, 2011 by Biblica, Inc.™ Used by permission of Zondervan. All rights reserved worldwide. www.zondervan.com The "NIV" and "New International Version" are trademarks registered in the United States Patent and Trademark Office by Biblica, Inc.™

Scripture quotations noted (NLT) are taken from the Holy Bible, New Living Translation, copyright ©1996, 2004, 2007, 2013, 2015 by Tyndale House Foundation. Used by permission of Tyndale House Publishers, Inc., Carol Stream, Illinois 60188. All rights reserved.

Scripture quotations noted (ESV) are from the ESV® Bible (The Holy Bible, English Standard Version®),copyright © 2001 by Crossway, a publishing ministry of Good News Publishers. Used by permission. All rights reserved.

Acknowledgements:

Jennifer Maly of Paper Lions Australia for proofreading and editing this book and Steve Blizzard for assisting Jennifer.

Cover art and direction by Shea Walsh

Typesetting & Printing by Images on Paper (WA) Pty Ltd

10/64-66 Kent Street, Cannington WA 6107

Contents

HOW TO BUILD A REHAB

If you do what you have always done,
you will just keep getting the same results.

FOREWORD

Over a decade ago, Peter Lyndon-James started Shalom House as a discipleship program with 6 men. Today, Shalom House now supports over 150 men and women (with children) in their journey of healing from addiction and rehabilitation. Focusing on the 'big picture,' Peter's third book, "How to Build a Rehab," has been written to assist local communities seeking to develop their own rehab program for those in need.

I first met Pete at a Men's Ministry when South African Farmer turned Evangelist, Angus Buchan led a series of men's meetings in Western Australia. At the time, a group of local men felt it was time to put a stop to the decline in society and turn things around. They decided to step up, taking personal responsibility for leading their families and making a difference in their community.

Following on from this, a series of men's 'Shed' Nights developed that continues to this day through Shalom House. Not long after this, Pete opened his original Shalom discipleship house.

As I got to know Pete, it became obvious we had come from very different sides of the track. Covered in tattoos, I learned that Peter had been a real wild child, becoming a Ward of the State as a young boy. In stark contrast, I had been raised in a supportive, extended farming family, becoming a Christian at a very early age while attending Northam Senior High School. As a result, I had never been drunk, never used drugs, was tattoo-free, had built a successful multi-million-dollar investment/insurance business, and was happily married with 3 children. I was the typical 'geek' that Pete wanted to become.

It is said that if you think someone doesn't have any personal struggles, you don't know them well enough. While I came from a relatively 'normal' family, the reality was that my mother suffered from bipolar disorder which led to my parent's divorce when I was 18. On the surface, having lived through the disruption of having a manic-depressive mother, it all made complete sense to me that they would go their separate ways. Unfortunately, it didn't take away the hurt after the event.

As a teen impacted by divorce, it feels like your family has been 'nuked' and you can become very self-reliant. My parents' divorce felt like being in a car and seeing a brick wall in front of you which you eventually hit. After everything fell apart, I ended up moving away from my family and charting my own course in life.

Pete ran some Men's camps on the South Coast from 2012 onwards, and then he took me along to a group course where I was able to go back and unpack the trauma of my parents' divorce that I had managed to bury deep within. Then in my late 40's, going back 30 years to unpack the trauma I had never dealt with, I was regarded as a 'hard case' by our group leader. The trauma was buried so deep, I had no idea it was a real problem. After a massive breakthrough, an immense peace came over me which led to an amazing renewal within my marriage and a massive improvement in how I related to my father and (now late) mother. I also discovered why my parents were the way they were. Without Pete's careful guidance, I wouldn't have experienced such incredible healing within my marriage and extended family.

Like my life changing-event, Pete's life was also miraculously turned around. Having worked alongside Pete as a long-term Volunteer Mentor within Shalom House, I know he is the real deal. Cheeky and tough as nails, Pete has an absolute heart of gold with an incredibly deep love for the families Shalom is helping to heal.

Following his time working as a Volunteer Prison Chaplain, Pete realised that the Justice system wasn't working, and he then developed the successful Shalom House program, as he knew what it would take to turn men (and women) around.

As I continued with my involvement with the Men's Shed night, I became a Volunteer Mentor within the program. Being privileged to mentor hundreds of men with Shalom over the past decade, I am now involved with leading group sessions and individual 'troubleshooting' mentoring. But none of this would have happened if Pete hadn't helped me to turn my life around first.

Being involved with Shalom can be like working in an Emergency Department. It can be confronting and sometimes sadly, it can be tragic. We recently celebrated Father's Day, and it was a real joy over the day to see countless Shalom graduates (now around the world) who were sharing their photos on social media of being fully restored to their families, with happy children blessed with a changed Dad (or Mum). This is what Shalom is all about.

"How to Build a Rehab" is more than a 'how-to' manual. I have personally witnessed that it is a tried and proven cutting-edge program that really works. Family after family, the Shalom House program is resulting in amazing outcomes that, without a doubt, will impact generations to come.

INTRODUCTION

Running a rehabilitation centre would have to be the hardest thing I have ever done with my life. I cannot count the number of days where I would go home at nighttime and lay on my bed, cuddling my pillow and crying as I rocked side to side, telling my wife that this was too much for me. It's hard to watch people make choices that not just affect themselves but also those they love. You can see that they have so much potential yet when they get to a certain point, they think that they are ready and try to move on and within weeks, they have not only lost everything that they worked towards, but again, hurt everyone that they love. Sorry can be a very powerful word but when it's used time and time again for the same thing, it loses its power.

One of the lessons that I learned in the first few years running Shalom was never to get emotionally attached. There have been a few residents over the years that I got emotionally attached to as I saw them grow through the program and their lives change. They got off drugs, managed to get debt free, repaired relationships with families and a couple of them even started small businesses through the program. But through a series of silly choices, they lost everything and went back to drugs, the toll that this can have on you personally if you don't set boundaries is huge. So I say never to get emotionally attached to any of those that you are trying to help as it may take you out in the process when things go wrong.

I don't come from an educated background and only ever made it to Grade Six in primary school, I'm not one to read books or study, I would rather just put my hand to something and work it out along the way. I have been that way my whole life. Being multi-skilled, I would build a structure, say a shed or trailer and then put together the documentation that I needed to support it together after or along the way. That's pretty much the same as Shalom House and how its whole program was put together.

Having spent my life in children's homes, on the streets, ward of the state, foster families, prisons, in and out of courts, on parole and being addicted to something most of my life all came to use in putting Shalom House's Holistic Model of Rehabilitation together. I spent 31 years on the wrong side of the fence doing the wrong things then my life turned around at the age of 31 when I became a Christian. At 32, I studied three years full-time theology at Riverview Bible College and then went on to work three days per week at Acacia Prison as a prison Chaplain for just on five years. The five years at Acacia Prison taught me a great deal. I saw the same prisoners coming in and then going out only to come back in again, the jail was not working but rather, it was making them worse. In prison you must project an image that people perceive to fit into where you are, kindness in prison is seen as a weakness, if you don't project the right image, you soon get put in your place. I saw the prison population explode in 2005 to 2010 from 400 to 1200, now today it sits on around 1900 plus prisoners, that's very sad but it wasn't just that prison but all the prisons.

In 2010, I finished at Acacia Prison and became a full-time volunteer trying to help whoever I could, wherever I could. For the next two and a half years. I helped many people on the streets get into rehabilitation centres, I volunteered at drug clinics, served at homeless shelters and assisted many ex-prisoners get help not to mention began hosting and facilitating men's camps and awareness groups. It seemed to me that no matter what I did I felt like I was chasing my tail, nothing seemed to be working, every day was like Groundhog Day. I couldn't understand why lives weren't changing, I honestly couldn't understand why it was that we all seemed to be chasing our tails trying to help people and it seemed like everybody that I did help was a waste of time. Some people would listen, and they might go good for a while and then I would plug them into a service that I felt could help them but in fact derailed them.

So in 2012 I drove passed a house not far from where I lived, and the house had a for sale sign on it so I went and looked at it and it felt right that it would work as a mentor house or should I say rehabilitation centre so I mortgaged my home and bought the house and then started Shalom House. I originally started with four residents that overtime went to seven, then to nine and it kept increasing. I never advertised but it was like I felt I was the pied piper who never played a pipe. Over the next few years, we went from the nine fellas to thirty then to seventy to one hundred and forty plus fellas across multiple properties.

Over the years I had to learn about the program, how to not just develop it, but also implement it as well as delegate it. People always used to say to make sure the program does not evolve around me or my personality, today I believe it runs not because of me but in spite of me. I learned Stage One and then developed Stage Two while at that same time working how the two stages can work together. Once I had stages one and two developed and implemented, I developed and implemented Stage Three making sure that it ran well with Stages One and Two and in the process, I continued with Stages Four and Five also being developed which finally ended with a graduation ceremony of the program after Stage Five.

In short, that's how the program came together, a five stage program that ends with a graduation. What is different about the program is our holistic approach to not just rehabilitation but also to reintegration and re-socialisation, we have everyone on the same page from the beginning of the program to the end of the program.

I was caught up in the government system my whole life, I call it the matrix, I don't mean to be rude, disrespectful or judgmental in saying that. Everyone who tried to help me over the course of my life tried to help in the best way that they knew how but sadly the work that one organisation did was undone by the work of the next organisation as they did it differently. There was no communication between the two organisations or they were not on the same page in regard to assisting myself hence going around in circles.

I have stolen cars, broken into homes, been in high speed chases, lived on the streets my whole childhood, spent time in jail, had a gun to my head, sold guns and drugs, been based and bashed and a lot whole heap more but I can honestly say with all my heart that I have received more hatred, death threats, lies told about me, legal problems and persecution trying to do the right thing on a weekly basis than I ever did doing the wrong thing. I feel like I have been run over by a road train, the last twelve and a half years has taken its toll on me personally but when I look back over the last ten years and see all the good Shalom has done in changing lives and restoring families and continues to do so today, I can honestly say that I would not change a thing.

If you look at the diagram on the next page, it would be fair to say that the CEO's position would be that of a facilitator of other services.

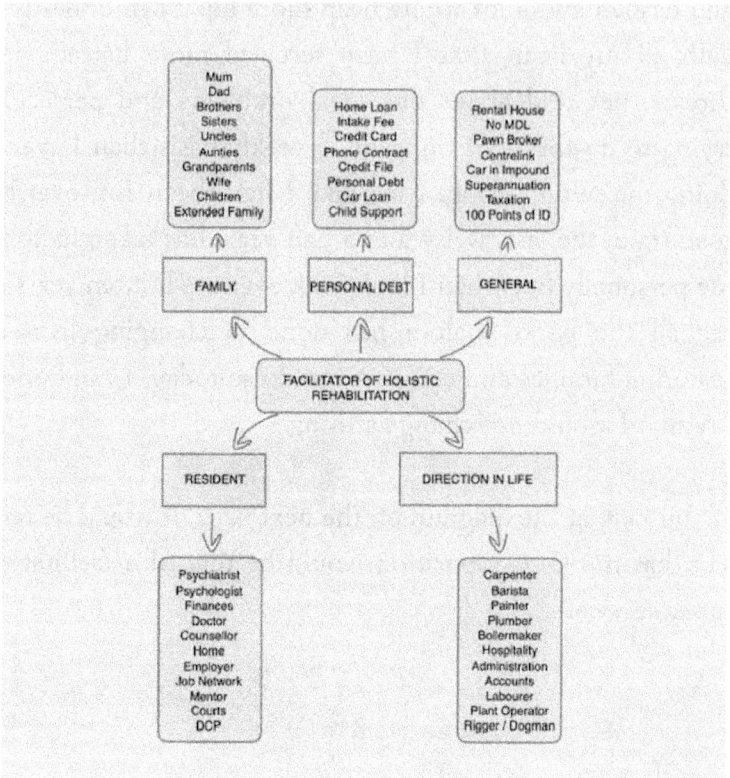

CHAPTER ONE — ABOUT ME

My name is Peter Lyndon-James. I have spent 26 years of my life in and out of children's homes, jails and institutions starting from the age of seven, and have a criminal record longer than most. I've broken into houses, stolen cars and mugged many people. I've sold drugs and guns, had genital warts, gonorrhea, crabs, herpes and more. Have I given it to others? Yes. Intentionally? No. I've played doctors and nurses as a child. I've fondled another boy's genitals growing up and I've also been sexually molested by a male as a child when I was 8. I have slept with many prostitutes behind my wife's back as well as with many other women.

For most of my life, I never paid taxes until I became a Christian. I, Peter Lyndon-James, have done all of the above and more. If it's not on there, I have probably done it.

Over the last 20 years on my journey to change my life, I have made many mistakes and still, like most of us, I have a long way to go. I have smoked pot a couple of times, smoked cigarettes, went back to alcohol, bought a firearm for fear of safety, used Methamphetamines, slept with another woman then had to tell my wife, and more. I did not change overnight.

All I can say is that if you are a victim of my life or my choices, if you are a victim of my selfishness and stupidity, I am sorry, I am so very sorry.

I have no excuse for what I have done to you or to any other person, what I have done was and is wrong and I am 100 percent to blame, there is nothing I can say in my defence.

Please, I ask that you would forgive me as I am genuinely sorry for my actions and wish I could change what I have done as well as the life I have lived, but I can't. All I can do is take ownership of my mistakes and try my best not to do it again. Today I really care about people. That other person is not me anymore, that person is dead, that's the old me. Today I am trying my best to be the best ME I can be. I care about people; I care about them in the way I need to, not in the way they want me to.

I don't care if you or any person on the face of this planet likes me, not even the slightest. But I do care what God thinks of me. I welcome any person to look over my life including my finances.

If there are areas in me or what I do that aren't done with honesty, integrity and transparency, then help me see what I can't see, for me to make the changes that I need to make. I am trying my best, please help me to be better.

THE WORD SHALOM MEANS
People ask me what the word Shalom means and where I got the name from. According to Strong's Concordance 7965, Shalom means: Completeness, Wholeness, Health, Peace, Welfare, Safety, Soundness, Tranquility, Prosperity,

Perfectness, Fullness, Rest, Harmony, as well as the absence of agitation or discord. Shalom comes from the root verb "shalom" meaning to be complete, perfect and full.

For me, it means to be complete, whole and full in every area of my life. It's the fullness of everything that is perfectly pure and good such as love, joy, peace, patience, kindness, goodness, gentleness, meekness, family, truth, transparency and integrity.

The word Shalom represents everything that I ever aspired to be. When the residents come into Shalom, they come in broken and at the end of themselves, so our goal for each resident is Shalom, to be the best US we can be, so we begin with the end in mind.

WHEN SHALOM FIRST STARTED

When I first started Shalom, I honestly did not have any intention of starting a rehabilitation centre. I just wanted to help people change their life like I had changed mine. I did not ask to grow up the way that I did and there are millions of kids like me. My whole life, all I wanted to be was a geek, a normal person, a productive member of society, to go to one school, not 16.

I only made it to Grade 6. I wanted to be able to run up the corridor in the morning to jump into bed with Mum and Dad for a cuddle, to go on family holidays, to play sports, to have friends and do normal stuff like normal families did, but sadly, it was completely the opposite for me.

I was put into children's homes from the age of seven and put in a boy's prison at nine. I spent my whole childhood either locked up in Longmore or Riverbank juvenile prisons or living on the streets in Perth from when I was 9 to 18 years old.

I was molested by a male at the age of nine and was also made a ward of the state. I became institutionalised. I have spent time in nearly every major adult prison in Western Australia: Hakea/Canningvale, Casuarina, Bunbury, Karnet and Wooroloo.

I consider my family to be those I grew up with: the drug addict, the criminal, the homeless person, the rejected and abandoned, the little boy who wanted Mum and Dad. My whole life, all I ever wanted was to be a normal person. I became a Christian in 2001. At the time, I was selling two and a half kilos of Methamphetamines a day as well as guns. My life has changed since then. I had to spend 12 years focusing on myself and changing my life, not just for me, but for my wife and children. I had to relearn how to be a man, a husband, a father. I literally had to learn everything that I wanted to be from scratch and my gosh, did I make many mistakes along the way.

A BRIEF TIMELINE

1970 — 1977

I was with Mum and Dad, moved around a bit and started school at Lockridge Primary School. Mum and Dad split up, Dad went up north and Mum started moving around all over the place.

1977 — 1987

I was made a ward of the state and was in and out of children's homes and foster families. I spent seven years in and out of Longmore Juvenile Prison for kids up to the age of 16, then I went to Riverbank from 16 until I was 18. When I was not in custody, I would live rough on the streets in Perth.

1987 — 1989

I met the mother of my daughter, Tosha-Lena, but I was always in trouble with the police, running from state to state or around Western Australia.

1989 — 2002

I was placed in an adult jail in 1991 and over the next eleven years, I kept moving around Australia, running from myself but wherever I went, I went. I have spent time in most of the prisons in Western Australia with my last prison term beginning in 2001.

2001 — 2005

I became a Christian in 2001 and went back to prison for minor charges and upon being released from jail, I enrolled in full-time Bible studies at Riverview Bible College.

I completed three years full-time study achieving Certificate IV in Ministry, Diploma of Theology and an Advanced Diploma in Theology.

2005 — 2010

In 2005, I started to volunteer three days a week as an ecumenical Prison Chaplain at Acacia Prison. Over my 5 years in Acacia Prison as a Chaplain, I kept seeing the same faces come in and go out. I also saw the prison population triple in size. When you get put in prison, you must project an image that people perceive to fit in with where you are. Kindness in prison is seen as a weakness.

You can take the prisoner out of prison, but then you must get the prison out of the prisoner.

One of the problems is that when you get placed into that environment or culture for one, two or three years, you have learned to project an image you need to fit in where you are, and you adapt to the culture.

When you are released from prison, I believe you are still in prison. It's hard mixing with normal people doing normal things as you feel like you don't fit in, that they are better than you, so you hang around people who make you feel comfortable, but the problem is that they are doing the exact things that you don't want to do anymore.

2010 — 2012
When I left the prison, I spent two and a half years floating around the streets and various rehabilitation centres in Perth, trying to find out what was working and what was not and all I saw was what I witnessed in the prison system. We were taking people off illegal drugs just to put them on legal ones. We were taking Heroin addicts off Heroin and putting them on Methadone, etc. Most addicts know strategies about how to tell a doctor or psychiatrist whatever they need to hear to get what they want or what makes them feel comfortable without them experiencing any real change in their lives. They would be chained to a chemist where they had to go daily to get their $7 a day dose.

2012 — 2022
In July of 2012, I started Shalom House and have spent the last twelve plus years trying to implement all I have learned to help others change their life like I have changed mine. I want them to experience the life that I now live, and it's working. In the beginning, I did not mean to start a rehabilitation centre, I was just discipling, or should I say mentoring people on how they could change their lives.

Over the next few years, I developed a five-stage program that is honestly working on not just the lives of men, but also women, children and families in our community. I know that there is no holistic program like this anywhere that is 100% self-funded and costs no one anything other than a few kind words and a bit of encouragement.

All I want is to make a difference in a positive way to as many lives as possible. It's sad to say, but I have received more hate, abuse and death threats in my life doing the right thing than I used to receive doing the wrong thing. It really doesn't make sense. I used to break the law and get lots of attention and now I am doing the right thing but cannot get any attention.

Shalom House is "Leading the way in Holistic Rehabilitation".

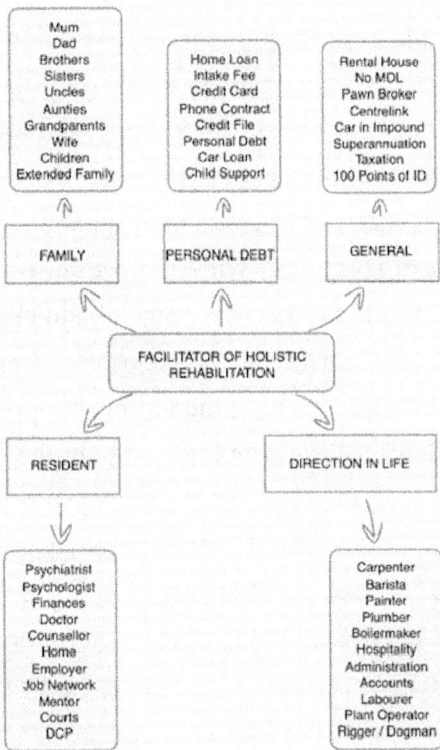

Mum	Home Loan	Rental House
Dad	Intake Fee	No MDL
Brothers	Credit Card	Pawn Broker
Sisters	Phone Contract	Centrelink
Uncles	Credit File	Car in Impound
Aunties	Personal Debt	Superannuation
Grandparents	Car Loan	Taxation
Wife	Child Support	100 Points of ID
Children		
Extended Family		

FAMILY — **PERSONAL DEBT** — **GENERAL**

FACILITATOR OF HOLISTIC REHABILITATION

RESIDENT — **DIRECTION IN LIFE**

Psychiatrist	Carpenter
Psychologist	Barista
Finances	Painter
Doctor	Plumber
Counsellor	Boilermaker
Home	Hospitality
Employer	Administration
Job Network	Accounts
Mentor	Labourer
Courts	Plant Operator
DCP	Rigger / Dogman

25

CHAPTER TWO — WHY HOLISTIC REHABILITATION?

I believe that it is important to have everyone on the same page when it comes to helping a person to not only change their lives and learn the skills to sustain the change, but also to deal with all of life's controlling issues, not just drugs and alcohol, especially when it comes to residential rehabilitation as most of the residents are struggling with more than one issue. These include heart/emotional issues, a range of addictions, childhood trauma, finances, separation or divorce, decision making, handling conflict, work ethics, mental health, criminal charges, government identification processes and employment.

By having the Counsellor, Doctor, Psychiatrist, Psychologist, DCP, Courts, Mentor, Job Network, Employer, Home Life all on the same page and with weekly communication by all involved, it helps everyone to work as a team in the best interests of those that they assist.

I have personally been a part of a broken system from the age of seven, where everyone involved in making any decisions about my life, deciding how to help as well as what to do were on different pages. This played a major part in me taking the wrong turns in life. This system makes it impossible for any effective, long-lasting rehabilitation to take place because all stakeholders have a different viewpoint and you just get caught up in the system, something I call the Matrix.

I know that everyone who ever tried to help me meant their best, but sadly, the ones who did a good job helping me had their work undone by someone else who went about what they did differently, from another perspective according to their beliefs, values and goals set by their employer/organisation. There are also many factors to take into consideration as I could relate to some people in my life and some I could not.

I had many people who were fresh out of high school or university making life-changing decisions on my behalf who had no lived experience, decisions that dramatically altered the course of my life. I had some professionals making decisions for me, giving me a range of solutions on how to fix my life while theirs was a total mess. These people had come from a place of lived experience and found a way out without properly dealing with their own issues.

They felt all fixed because they survived, so they did a counselling course and then went on to try to help others but ended up unintentionally hurting their clients. Please don't be offended by what I say as you read this book. I'm not wanting to have a go at anyone but rather, work together as a team to continue to implement what works as it can be taken so many different ways. I'm sure if we did work together then our outcomes would be much greater.

Depending on the issues that are identified and their severity, this would lead us to decide who needs to be involved.

Also, by working as a team, it would highlight the departments that cross over in their roles ensuring clear collaboration by all.

The smaller the issue, then fewer people would need to be involved. The greater the issue, then the need is higher for a coordinated approach using people with the right skill sets who can work together as one to deal with the issues.

It's imperative that the rehabilitation centres communicate with the doctors, counsellors, mental health services, psychologists, psychiatrists, courts, lawyers, community services, Relationships Australia, Department For Child Protection (DCP), families, employers and schools.

All parties need to be on the same page with facilitated communication being the best possible outcome for those they are helping but sadly, this is often not the case.

I know that many people would say that it is simply not possible, but I would disagree as that is exactly what we do here at Shalom. The only struggle we face now is with the justice system and enablers but apart from that, we have everyone on the same page regarding each individual, a truly holistic rehabilitation.

We have had residents in Shalom for eighteen months or more where their families were restored, they were working full-time, free from all drugs and substances, only to have them sent to jail on old charges. It's very sad because in most of these cases,

I can confidently say that their lives have been changed for the better. Yes, they deserve punishment for their crimes, but isn't the ultimate objective of incarceration rehabilitation?

It's important that medical professionals communicate with each other on a weekly basis and share what it is that they see as well as what the next step forward might be. This is so we can all act as one moving forward in the best interests of those we are trying to assist. It's extremely important that we break down what we see and break it into small outcomes in chronological order (meaning start from the basics) with the main objective being a fully changed life in all areas.

Every stakeholder does their best to help, but unfortunately, when other organisations or health professionals do things differently, all that good work might come undone for someone not suited to that style. If another organisation does it differently again, it just goes around in circles. These are people's lives we are talking about, I know we don't want them to go in circles but I believe that's what's happening.

LEADING THE WAY IN HOLISTIC REHABILITATION
There is not a program like Shalom House anywhere else in Australia, achieving the results we are, it's a highly specific model. It's astounding: 100% self-funded and all our residents are off Centrelink benefits within 4-7 months after entering the program as they are working back in the working community.

The residents are being productive members of society while at the same time, they are developing life skills and positive coping mechanisms to sustain the changes that they have made in their lives.

Taking a holistic approach to rehabilitating a person's life may not be for everyone because of the length of commitment involved. Those who decide to take that path and who can finish what they started will achieve more in a short time than they probably would over a lifetime. Imagine being able to put aside twelve to eighteen months of your life just to focus on yourself.

To be able to:
- Clean up your heart issues
- Work at restoring all family relationships
- Learning financial independence
- Being 100% debt free
- Having all your taxation and superannuation completed and up to date
- Obtaining a full-time job
- Getting a driver's licence
- Purchasing a car
- Having your own rental and owning your own furniture
- Developing good communication skills
- Knowing how to deal with the pressures of life
- Having good conflict resolution skills
- Knowing how to maintain and complete everyday tasks such as cook, clean etc.

Basically, our Holistic Rehabilitation program covers every area of a person's life. Through the program, not only do they clean their past up, they slowly learn to fix it, and they also learn the skills they need to learn to lay the foundation to maintain what they have received.

STAGES OF ADDICTION

You can class a person's stage of addiction by using the following categories. It is made up of seven stages: A, B, C, D and E but there are actually three types of E's. Now depending on what stage a person is at determines which course of action you would take to help that person.

Class A

A — is a person who is first starting on the pathway to drugs. A young person who is hitting the age of between eleven to fifteen going okay at school, but is facing the challenges of puberty, home life, identity etc. and asking themselves where they fit in. They might have been bullied at school that day or had an argument at home then he/she goes out to a party and sees a heap of other kids having a good time, one of them is smoking cones or drinking alcohol, and the young person gets offered one. Before they try the drug, inside their head, one voice says, "Go on, have one, everyone else is doing it," with another voice saying, "Don't be stupid, you know it's wrong."

Often, with a bit of peer pressure, the young person makes the wrong choice, and they try it. Remember the first time that you had your first beer, cone or even cigarette? Depending on the individual and the effects it has on them, this will determine if they continue its use. There are many people who have a very bad experience the first time they use drugs and vow never to do it again. There are also many who love the euphoria the drugs or substances gives them and finds a new sense of purpose and strength to fit in, something that they never had before.

Our experience at Shalom House has been that many of my fellas who were at that stage were facing problems at home or something had happened to them that they couldn't or wouldn't talk to anyone about. We have had many fellas who have experienced bullying as a child, they have never really fitted in with the cool kids. Then one day they go to a party and the cool kids were using drugs, and with a bit of pressure, they tried some and found a level of acceptance from their peers that they never had before, encouraging them down the wrong path. They go home the next day, and they feel guilty for what they did. They know that it was wrong but don't want to get into trouble.

One voice says, "Tell your mum or dad," and the other voice says, "No it's OK, you didn't hurt anyone." They decide to keep what they did to themselves, not knowing that they have just planted the seeds of addiction, lies, deceit and a whole lot more. That's typical of A's the first time they used drugs or substances and they also found that the drug or the substance covered up the anger and other negative emotions that they were feeling.

Class B

B — is someone who has tried drugs or substances the first time, thought to themselves that they didn't hurt anyone and had kept it to themselves. For a few days after the first time, they felt a little convinced that they should tell their parents but now that conviction had gone away.

They get invited to a party the following week so they go along and one of the cool kids from the week before is there and they get offered a cone or a drink.

Their first voice says, "Don't do it, you're mad," while the other voice in their head says, "Go on, you didn't hurt anyone, remember?"

The child thinks about it and reflects on the week just gone and thinks, "That's right, I didn't hurt anyone." They see no harm in it, as "Everyone else is doing it." They say to themselves, "I'm not hurting anyone, it's no different than mum or dad having a beer." That's a B, they have now accepted that it's OK, it's the social thing to do. The excuses begin. Every weekend, they make it the standard norm to go out with their mates, have a few cones or drinks. B's are pretty hard to turn around or talk to as they see no harm in what they are doing. They have made their choice, "It's okay," they say. The euphoria that the drug or alcohol gives you far outweighs the guilt of making wrong choices. Deception starts at A and settles into the heart here at B. If a person believes a lie as truth, that lie becomes THEIR truth.

Class C

C — is someone who just doesn't listen. They say, "I only do it on weekends. I'm not hurting anyone. It's only Fridays and Saturdays. It's only every fortnight. I'm okay."

.

But over time, the use escalates to a point where they can't stop if they tried. Cones are now a thing of the past, with meth (ice) or hammer (heroin) more often being the drug of choice at this stage. Weekly usage now moves to daily, there's no stopping them now. They have made a conscious choice to go down the path they are taking. They wind down at the end of the day by having a few cones, a couple of beers and have started trying other drugs. Marijuana cones are the standard norm during the week, and the heavier drugs are the weekend delight. The same cycle continues except now with the heavier drugs.

Slowly, the identity of the person starts to change, the friends they have, the way they talk. You can see the person changing and you start to have suspicions that things aren't quite the same, but you can't put your finger on it. You approach the individual to raise some of your concerns, but they come up with an explanation you accept as reasonable, but deep down, you know it's not. They start to become unreliable, taking longer to do certain tasks, asking for short-term loans from family and friends, talking a lot more than they used to and showing symptoms of paranoia. The stages of C's & D's are the most destructive, not just on the person, but also on the families and others involved, both directly and indirectly.

Class D

D — There's no stopping a D as the use of drugs is now daily, with the heavier drugs being the drug of choice. People around them can see them changing, and yet the user themselves is blinded to the changes taking place inside them. If they were not blinded, they would not refuse to look or listen to people who point out the obvious to them.

Everything about them is changing, the way they speak, the way they treat those around them. Their morals and values aren't the same anymore, their priorities and the people they are hanging around, everything. Financially, they are starting to fall apart, loans and bills are not getting paid on time, they start to ask family members for small loans, making excuses why they need the money and are continually having to cover their tracks as to why.

Their use of drugs starts to get so bad they are missing work because they did not wake up in time, and when they are at work, the quality of their output is no longer the same. The employer sees a massive change in the addict, with their ability to cope and get work done in the workplace no longer being there. Their moods are so bad now it seems that everyone in the home must tiptoe around on eggshells so as not to upset the drug-affected family member.

People can clearly see the drug's effects on a D and they try to bring truth to the user, but the user will not have a bar of it. They consider it an attack and start to blame the person bringing the truth to them. The user blames the messenger for the circumstances that they are in and somehow, it gets turned back on the person trying to help. The user blames you or others for the way that they are, no matter what you say, they think the addict is not at fault.

What is really saddening is that families honestly only know 10 percent of what is going on and are left to give advice, knowing very little of what is really happening. As you can tell, all of this usually takes place over a few years depending on the individual, their family life, their finances etc.

Class E

E — Everything has come to a head, the person has lost their job, been kicked out of home, or has been forcibly removed from the home by police and restraining orders have been put in place. The addict's bills can no longer be paid as their source of funds has finally dried up. The family support has stopped because their financial resources have been exhausted. The user is at the bottom of the bottom of the bottom. They ring relatives up, crying for help, saying they are ready to change, they finally admit that they need help and tell their family members everything they want to hear, but it's just so the addict can get what they want, not really willing to change. What the E says answers a whole heap of questions you had plus confirms your presumptions. Again, the series of stuff that unfolds depends on each person's circumstances and background.

ENABLING

What I see quite often with an E is the wife, for example, has had enough. Husband is an E, he has hit the wall and the wife has been brought to the point where she has no choice but to have hubby forcibly removed from the home. So, Mum and Dad, in their stupidity, try to step in and intervene by bringing their son back into their home and everything that happened under his wife's roof continues to happen under his parents' roof. The cycle then continues again except that because of the break and a new roof over his head, he has now dropped back to a C or a D. Because of the parents' lack of insight as to what he has been up to, he brings his bad stuff to their home and then his bad stuff over time spreads onto them. They start to experience what the wife went through and over time, he picks up drugs and becomes an E again.

Finally, Mum and Dad must have the E removed from the property. One of the problems is that after he has gone or been removed from the property, the marriage between the two parents is never the same again. This is because Mum and Dad end up with unforgiveness and bitterness in their hearts towards each other as well as towards their son. Mum said to do it this way and Dad said to do it that way, it brings massive amounts of division into the family unit, with some marriages never recovering.

The three types of E's

E1 — Hits the brick wall and they will do whatever they can to change their lives.

E2 — Swaps an illegal addiction for a legal one, prescription medication. They swap the Heroin for the Methadone or the meth for prescription medication.

E3 — This type of E is the ones we build jails for. They are quite happy doing what they are doing and have no genuine desire to stop what they are doing and change their lives for the better. They are also the original reason why prisons were built, to punish a person for their crimes.

How you help an A is different to how you help a B. You cannot help a C or a D in the way that you want to but you must help them in the way that they need you to. Out of the three E types of addicts, we only take in the E1's here at Shalom. The other two types of E's are not suited to our model of Holistic Rehabilitation. If you were to take them in and mix the three E's together, then it would work against what we are trying to achieve here at Shalom.

In one of my other books, "Tough Love, Tackling Drug Addiction & Seeing Change," it will show you how to help the A's, B's, C's and D's as well as the three E's and much more. It will also show you what you NEED to do and not what you WANT to do.

The first decision to make is the decision to change your life, that's the ideal outcome for every family. Wouldn't it be easy if everyone automatically made that choice? But in reality, for C's & D's, it's very unlikely and for the E's, it can be a strong possibility depending on how the individual families handle it.

What I find is that most families think they are doing the right thing, but in actual fact, they are doing the wrong thing.

In that case, a person may stay caught up in addiction many years longer than they should have.

I want the E's to come to me at Shalom House, as long as there are no other options such as mum's, dad's or in-laws' house or mates. I can help the E's, but I need all of the E families to help.

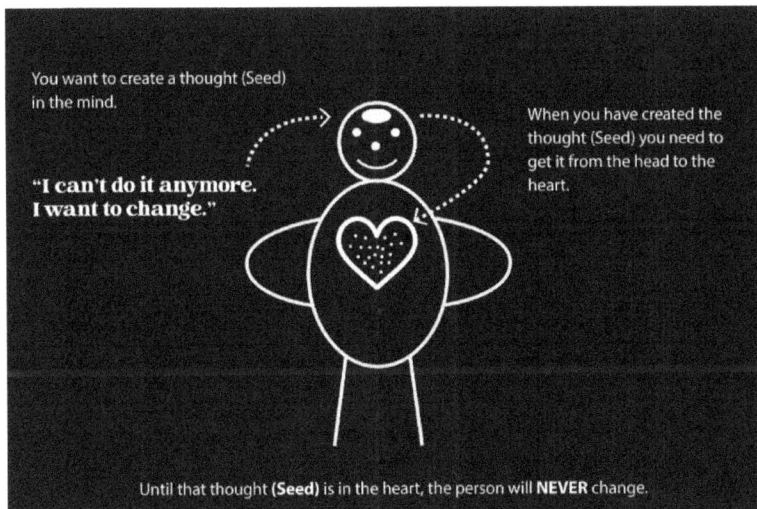

You want to create a thought (Seed) in the mind.

"I can't do it anymore. I want to change."

When you have created the thought (Seed) you need to get it from the head to the heart.

Until that thought (Seed) is in the heart, the person will NEVER change.

Somehow, I need to get their mind thinking, "I can't do this anymore, I want to change."

When the mind creates that thought, which I call a seed, "I can't do this anymore," and then the person makes their mind up, it becomes "I want to change," where that seed goes from the HEAD to the HEART.

When they come and see me, I can tell if that seed is there in the heart during my intake process. I can water that seed, I can make it grow into a changed life.

I know how to make it grow, that's good. Once the seed is there, then begins the process of cleaning up the heart.

CHAPTER THREE — RESIDENTS PAY FOR THEIR OWN REHABILITATION

All the residents pay for their own rehabilitation, let me tell you why and then how. Many people who have never tried drugs don't understand why drugs are enjoyable, they can't stand the thought of it and can't comprehend why on earth people use them.

I used drugs for 26 years and enjoyed them, I loved the highs they gave me and the good times I had when I was on them, life became exciting, and they seemed to take away all my problems. I knew the serious consequences of using drugs as I had suffered them for years, but I didn't seem to care.

"Stuff the world." I thought, "I'm not hurting anyone."

I knew the risks, Hep C, bad health, financial ruin, family breakdowns and a whole heap more, but I didn't care. I was having fun and they seemed to take away my problems, or so I thought.

Shalom House is 100% self-funded and does not receive any financial support from the government or other agencies. Currently, we have 150 men, Women and Children in our facility across 13 houses and growing every month because the need is so high.

HOW WE ARE FUNDED

I charge each one of my residents $300 per week for full board and not a cent more. Out of that, we must pay the rents on 13 properties ($10,000 per week), utilities on the thirteen properties, feed and transport 150 men, women and children plus pay the wages of 50 plus staff, not to mention those who are a part of the couples' program and much more.

Again, I don't believe that society should have to pay to rehabilitate a drug user, it's not OK. They are the ones that had fun for many years getting stoned off their face, they are the ones who chose to use drugs, they should be the ones to pay for their own rehabilitation, not the taxpayer or another individual.

IT'S WORKING

We are wanting to raise awareness of what we are doing and to let people know that we believe that we have a program that is working and can be rolled out across Australia and beyond. It can be easily adapted to suit any organisation that will not only help people caught up in addiction, restore families, save billions of taxpayers' funds, help people struggling with mental health, transform the prison system, and more.

Yes, we are a registered tax-deductible charity that has deductible gift recipient (DGR) status as well as a Charitable Collections Licence. If it weren't for a few generous people who have given to Shalom, we would be doing it a lot harder than we are.

I try never to ask people for money but if they get prompted to give, they receive a tax-deductible receipt, and we make sure we use our funds wisely. Shalom also has a very functional board as well as an external auditor who goes over our books every year to ensure we are using our funds wisely and that every dollar is accounted for.

Another reason I write all this is that I would like to always be open, honest and transparent in all that I do. I welcome any individual or organisation to look at our books and ask any questions with regards to Shalom, Shalom Works or anything else that I may put my hand to. You will see that we are honest, accountable and are transparent in all that we do. It takes a great deal of commitment by everyone involved to make Shalom House work. From the staff to the volunteers and general public, it's a team effort. Many sacrifices have been made by all involved to get Shalom to where it is today. We are not about making money but focused on changing and transforming lives.

Shalom House is funded by those within the program, and in return, they get their whole life sorted out. We help them to bring, where possible, complete restoration to their entire family. We also bring restoration to all their finances and general issues, as well as set them up in a career of their choosing for their future. We are a Holistic Rehabilitation Centre that works at bringing complete restoration to the individual and in turn, flowing positivity into their families. Isn't that awesome?

It's not costing anyone anything except the person who has been using drugs, and even then, they still receive a lot more than what they give. I don't believe it's Ok for a person to wilfully use drugs and substances and have a lot of fun doing so, then when the consequences of their actions catch up with them, for them to just rock up at a government or non-government organisation and expect the taxpayer or another individual to pay for their rehabilitation. They are the ones who got themselves into their mess so they should be the ones to get themselves out of it and in turn, they learn in the process.

RESIDENT INTAKE PROCESSES

The first thing we need to do is to find out if the resident is ready for the program. I do this on the first day that I meet with them. They have no idea that when they come for their intake interview there is an exceptionally strong chance that they will come into the program then and there on the day, or not at all. But I will ask myself if they are an E1.

The reason I take them in without any notice given to any person is that I don't want them to go on a bender on drugs or to get blind drunk the night before. Also, many people who are used to the rehabilitation and prison systems know how to prepare themselves prior to going in. They think to themselves that this will be the last time for a long while, so they get smashed and go on a bender. Another way they prepare is by hiding drugs inside their body, either by swallowing it or inserting it you know where, I'm sure you can guess.

RESIDENT INTAKE

Part of the resident's intake will be to get them to do an induction into the program. This is where we explain the rules to the house, and what we do during the week as well as the weekends. We explain why we shave their heads, why we go to three different churches, why only one radio station, why they are paired up, what they're allowed and not allowed to have in the house. We also explain to them what days they can make phone calls, what happens on family nights as well as what we do for activities on the weekends, and how the house runs. We also explain to all new residents how to communicate with the office to get things done on their behalf through the communication slips that we have on all properties.

FAMILY INFORMATION

On intake with new residents, we explain to the family members how there will be no contact with the resident for the first couple of weeks. If families wish to get an update on how the resident is going, they can contact Resident Care. It's explained to the families that if they wish to bring items into the house for their loved one, they can do so by contacting Resident Care and obtaining approval. We also explain to all families how the program works, family days, phone calls, our weekly routine as well as what will happen when the Mentor contacts them.

PSYCHIATRIST

We are very grateful to Dr Willem Van Wyk for his long-term service to Shalom. He has been with us now for twelve years. Dr Willem visits Shalom on a weekly basis in a voluntary capacity. All residents who need to see Dr Willem on a professional basis do so with a GP referral at his office.

All new residents at Shalom see a qualified psychiatrist within the first 7 days, but if required, within 24 hours depending on the resident. If it is deemed necessary, the resident will see the psychiatrist on a weekly basis. Shalom follows Dr Willem's instructions to the letter regarding all medications. What he prescribes, we give.

DR WILLEM VAN WYK — PSYCHIATRIST

I asked Dr Willem a few questions about his time working with Shalom over the last twelve years and the following was his response.

"In short, life changing. It has changed my perspective a great deal. It is easy to have ideas and opinions about lots of things but to see what is possible and how things really work is a different thing altogether. Shalom is the ideal place of healing that I always aspired towards, and I imagine it could be the same for many others who see the helping profession as a vocation, not a career move or a popularity contest.

Every week after I have been to Shalom, I return to my day job with renewed inspiration and understanding. In the beginning, I thought I had useful skills and may be able to lend a helping hand with Shalom. It didn't take me long to realise that I was getting much more out of volunteering my services at Shalom than I was giving.

When I look back at how my own life has changed over the period that I have been involved with Shalom, it is humbling because I felt I have been through rehab myself. I am not the same person that I was or the same person that I might have been without Shalom, and that is no overstatement."

SHALOM'S REHAB MODEL AS SEEN FROM DR WILLEM VAN WYK's PERSPECTIVE

The main thing is that Shalom House's rehab model works, whatever explanation one would give for how or why it works. This is not just another one of the latest rehab models. I don't question the likelihood that each rehab model will have good aspects and that all of them will contribute to the betterment of society.

But if one looks for one model that stands out above the others — looking the gold standard in rehab — I suggest that people look at Shalom.

My understanding is that Shalom is set up as a mentorship model where residents are surrounded by mentors who have often been through similar experiences but have gone further down the recovery pathway, working their way through those issues. People often talk about client-centered practice and then do the opposite. Shalom truly puts the individual first. Add in mentorship to the equation and you get a person-centered approach for all involved in rehab rather than a complicated theoretical model. The strength of this approach is the quality of the people involved, not how good the theoretical model looks on paper or sounds at workshops/conferences.

Although every resident has their own program, the common denominator for all residents is the Christian way of life. Many non-Christians talk about their experiences in a Christian setting, and it is seldom a major issue since the Christian values have been built into Western civilisation for the past 2000 years. Christians are followers of Jesus and they are everywhere in society. Meeting more of these 'traditional/old school' people than one might otherwise would doesn't come as a surprise for most non-Christian residents I have spoken to.

Those who look for something to criticise at Shalom tend to focus on the topic of Christianity very quickly, but I have not seen one case where I felt Shalom got it wrong or that Christianity was inappropriate or harmful to any resident. Christianity is not a cult or a sect but Christians are a certain kind of person because of their commitment to live life a certain way — which also happens to be a healthy way.

I don't know a lot about the similarities and differences between other rehabs. What I do know is that Shalom is the most 'hardcore' rehab that I have come across. It sounds bad but when you discuss the issue of control with residents, they acknowledge that they need rigid structure to escape from the clutches of life-controlling situations.

Each rehab will draw a different population of people. My understanding is that there isn't one rehab that can cater for every addict's needs. If the other rehabs get people engaged in treatment or get their residents over the line into recovery, may God bless them too.

When you deal with the more severe end of the addiction spectrum, Shalom House's more rigid structure is, in my understanding, an essential part of being most effective. Once a person's life has become controlled by addictions and other life-controlling issues, it would be naive to imagine that a more liberal rehab could give them the freedom and hope they desire without initially delegating control of their lives to a trustworthy person or organisation. Gradually, they need to earn that control back. I routinely have this conversation with residents, some of whom have failed other rehab approaches, and they confirm this sentiment.

The Culture

It is vitally important that everyone needs to be on the same page and pull in the same direction. Pete has managed to build up and maintain a healthy culture through bold leadership and clear vision. The Christian way of life is not merely an organised religion or a set of rules but a certain (healthy) kind of person living a certain (healthy) kind of life. I am aware of several other ideologies in contemporary society but when you look at the kind of culture that is associated with other ideologies, Shalom stands head and shoulders above the others.

What To Expect

I am used to forming an idea of a person's prognosis in my day job—estimating what the chance is that the person may recover and how I imagine that may look. At Shalom, I have stopped doing that and say to people that I simply don't know what to expect from their recovery (what it may look like) but I will expect considerable change, based on what I have seen with others.

Every single Shalom resident surprise me when I look back after a few days, weeks, months or years as I could never have imagined what I see. I am aware that this kind of statement may appear overly dramatic when in fact, it is more likely to be understated than overrated. One must experience the enormity of change in the lives of residents, their families and loved ones to understand the significance. Because of the changes that I have seen in residents, I have learned not to put a lid on my expectations for potential recovery of even the worst of the worst, by the grace of God. What I can add, based on my observations is that the most dramatic, rapid and lasting change can be observed once people form a personal relationship with God; it is like the lights going on inside the resident.

Prescription Medication

I support Shalom House's preference to get people into rehab without non-essential medication and re-introduce medication down the track once if it is proven to be essential as based on the observable features of their physical or mental health rather than their feelings or preferences. While contemporary culture is much more permissive regarding use of non-essential chemicals, this approach is consistent with traditional good clinical practice.

What Shalom is good at:

- Relationships — with each other, family, community and with God
- Connectedness — belonging, fitting in, finding your place
- Tolerance — as rigid as Shalom's boundary conditions may appear, there is a far greater freedom and tolerance of disruptive and disordered behaviour than in a less supported environment
- Support — I heard a conversation between Peter and a senior leader where they agreed on the belief that you can never support a person too much. That was a novel idea for me, but I have come to understand how true it is. Pull the support away too soon and things go wrong.

- Certainty — people know exactly what Shalom stands for, what is OK and what is not OK. Freedom isn't the absence of boundaries but the safety within clear, predictable boundaries.
- Safety — safe places with safe people can be a rarity in contemporary life. I explicitly trust Peter and Shalom. Not that nothing can go wrong but when they do, they will be dealt with and become learning/growing experiences.

How To Improve

If I had ideas, I would say that, but I am not aware of any glaring issues. People are imperfect so there will always be a splinter to be found in the eyes of another. The day that Shalom is no longer working i.e., no longer helping people, I will have opinions on things to be improved.

All of these answers were in response to my questions to Psychiatrist Dr Willem Van Wyk.

DOCTOR

All residents on admission to Shalom House will see one of Shalom's GP's for an initial assessment within 24 hours where a full health check-up will take place, including bloods and urine. If medication is prescribed by the doctor, then we will follow their instructions as to its administration.

PRESCRIPTION MEDICATION

Please forgive me if it seems like I am having a go at medical professionals as I am not. I believe today that some hand out far too much prescription medication, especially to addicts. When you are an addict, you know how to tell any doctor what they need to hear to get what you want. I know that I used to explain my symptoms and tell the doctor whatever they needed to hear to get the drugs that I wanted.

Most medical professionals are obligated by law to prescribe the medication required depending on the symptoms a person displays and if they don't do so and something happens to that person, in some cases, they can be found to be liable. If the doctor I went to see did not give me what I wanted, I would continue to find other doctors until I got what I wanted. It was not hard.

Some prescription medications can take people from an illegal drug to a legal one. It's not hard to get addicted to prescription medication. You start with one pill a day then slowly begin to self-medicate by increasing the dosage. As long as the person gets a kick from the chemical, they feel they are fine but their tolerance levels begin to rise. In turn, so does their usage.

Some prescription medications are very strong, take Xanax for example. It comes in 2mg form and may look very small but my gosh, it packs a punch and for someone who has not had one before, it will knock you out cold. As you build up a tolerance to them, you need more to get that same effect. We have just detoxed a girl who was on 50 x 2mg pills per day, heroin, meth, plus whatever else she could find.

I AM NOT AGAINST PRESCRIPTION MEDS

I am not against prescription medication and believe that it's OK for people to take Schedule 8 (S8) medications for a short term if required, but not for extended periods of time. We really need to be cautious when giving prescription medication to addicts.

S8 medications should be highly restricted and limited in quantity: Clonazepam, Xanax, Diazepam, Hydrocodone, Methadone, Oxycodone, Ketamine, Fentanyl, Lyrica, Seroquel, Codeine, Temazepam, Serapax, Panadeine Forte, Endone, etc. They now say that 9.3 percent of Australians suffers with some type of depression, so they hand out antidepressants like lollies. What people are really struggling with are life issues such as anger, conflict, unforgiveness, guilt, shame, regret, trauma, rejection, lack of worth and self-esteem, to name a few.

Prescription medication is being used as a band-aid while not treating the root cause of the issue. Blood pressure, vitamins, antibiotics, etc. do not fall under the S8 category.

As I have mentioned, I am not against prescription medication but I believe that the first approach should be to try and deal with the issues you are struggling with and use these medications as a last resort. I have found that most medications seem to act as a wall or a band aid preventing you from dealing with the root cause of the issue. We do have qualified Doctors, a Psychiatrist, a Psychologist and Counsellors who are also in agreement with the above.

CHAPTER FOUR — MENTORS

All residents are assigned to a mentor who will be assigned to them for the duration of their stay. Mentors do change depending on their relatability to the residents. Having mentors helps the residents to unpack their daily struggles while in the program and to understand the tools needed to maintain the strong positive culture. Mentors will also assist the residents with any heart issues that may arise, plus mediate and facilitate between family members and loved ones during the reconciliation process.

DEVELOP A NORMAL ROUTINE

It's really important for all residents to develop a daily normal routine as soon as they enter the program as many residents, due to their addiction and bad choices, have no routine at all. From Monday to Friday, all residents should be out of bed by 6 am to clean their rooms and make their beds, have breakfast and get their lunch ready. Everybody across all properties and in all work parties and crews start their day around 8.30 am with a group devotional where we discuss scriptures and other related issues: dealing with offence, unforgiveness, honesty, family decision-making, etc.

Between 9 am and 4 pm, everybody is sent out to work, whether it be on the block, our main base, or in the office or even out on the work trucks carrying out tasks such as fencing, paving, mechanical duties, office administration, café/hospitality duties, maintenance, crews, furniture removal, farm work and more.

We generally finish work around 4 pm when everybody can return to their houses and have free time. Every Tuesday night, we have a Men's Night which runs from 6 pm to 9 pm. Every Wednesday night, the women have a Women's Night which runs from 6 pm to 9 pm. Every Friday night, we go to various churches throughout the city: the ladies to one church and the men to another. These services go from around 6 pm to 9 pm.

Saturday mornings across all properties mean major house cleans where we clean all properties from head to toe. The house cleaning usually finishes around 11 am and then all residents will go out on their daily activity, whether it be to the beach, a bushwalk, roller-skating, a movie or a barbecue in the park. The men will go one way and the ladies go another, with the activities alternating every weekend.

Every Saturday night is Family Night where we meet at the Blue Gum Community Centre. This is where all residents are allowed to invite their loved ones: mums and dads, children, partners, uncles, aunties and very close friends. This goes from 4:30 pm till 8 pm every Saturday. All families are encouraged to bring a plate of food to share during the night so we all have a meal together. The service itself starts at 5 pm until 6:30 pm followed by dinner and fellowship.

On Sundays, all residents have a sleep-in and need to be out of bed by 8 am and ready to head to church within the hour. Every weekend, we go to different church services and denominations across the city as I have explained previously.

After church on Sundays, all residents head to the shops to do their own personal weekly shopping and then return to the houses, having the remainder of the day to rest and have free time. That is our regular weekly routine, and the cycle begins again on Monday.

Get Work Ready
All residents from Day One of the program work from Monday to Friday 9 am to 4 pm. The types of work that they undertake depends on what's available. They will all start out working at the Men's or Ladies' block for the beginning of the program as we need to keep a close eye on them until they settle in which is farm or general labouring-type work. After four weeks, other opportunities become available. This could be on the trucks in the community, carrying out general garden maintenance or in the workshop, doing administration, cleaning up the properties or even in the café as this helps them to develop a regular routine and prepare them for Stage Two where they will be sent out to paid work starting at two days a week.

The entirety, meaning 100% of the income that they earn from paid work goes to the resident to be put into their trust fund. It generally takes around three months to prepare a resident to be work ready. Over that time, we have had much to deal with: counselling, reconciliation of relationships, developing a working routine, medical issues, dealing with finances, etc.

FAMILY SUPPORT

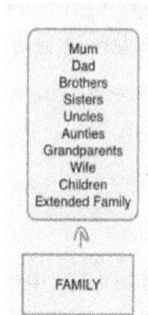

```
┌─────────────────────┐
│        Mum          │
│        Dad          │
│      Brothers       │
│       Sisters       │
│       Uncles        │
│       Aunties       │
│    Grandparents     │
│        Wife         │
│      Children       │
│   Extended Family   │
└─────────────────────┘
           ⇑
┌─────────────────────┐
│       FAMILY        │
└─────────────────────┘
```

NEW RESIDENT, PAUL

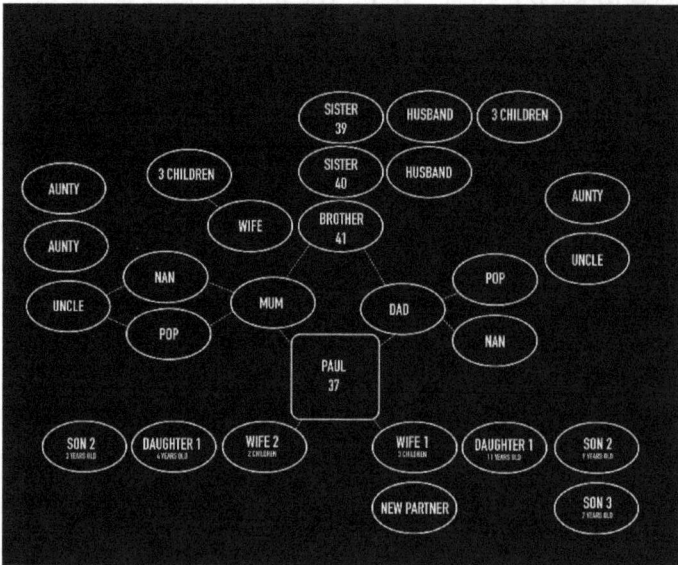

When a resident first comes in, they are all over the place emotionally. They keep reflecting on the damage they have done and the people they have hurt and "I don't know what to do," especially as they detox.

If you look at the specific resident Popplet example above, you can see that new resident Paul has two wives but his mind will be focused on his second wife and two children because he believes that he has done too much damage with his first wife. His first wife now has a new boyfriend and he hasn't seen his children from her in a long time.

So, we look at the Popplet, knowing that he would be missing his children from his second wife, but we also understand that his second wife needs a break from him so what we do is we will catch up with her mother or his mother and see where they sit in regard to their relationship with Paul.

If one of them is strong enough, then we will organise for that person to bring Paul's children in on Saturdays so he can see them at Family Night, and it starts from there. This creates a bit of hope in Paul and also helps him to focus on giving his best.

It's important to understand that every program is different, every family circumstance is unique, what's unfolding in their life is different to all other residents to date. It can't be one approach fits all, it doesn't work that way. Our goal for all residents over the course of their program would be to have every relationship restored with all friends and family. We carry out many reconciliations between the residents and their family members at different times depending on each person's circumstances.

Some family members are willing to engage in communication and others have had enough and "I don't want anything to do with the resident." Over time, they hear the stories about the changes that have taken place in the resident's life and it sparks curiosity and eventually we hope they will engage in the reconciliation process.

Having family relationships restored creates a lot of hope and builds momentum within every resident's life, thinking that "Maybe I can fix this."

We acknowledge that not all relationships will be restored, and that includes marriages. What we do hope to achieve is that we can get both parties on talking terms respectfully in the best interests of not just the children, but also other family and friends. We know that it takes a great deal of time to earn back the trust that they have lost due to the resident's actions.

CREATE CULTURE & ENVIRONMENT
In Shalom, we don't allow swearing, talking about drugs, crime or women in a negative way. We don't want a resident glorifying the past in any way, shape or form, it's regurgitating the memories of the past that limit the progress of the future. We help residents to deal with everyday issues that come up

such as lies, unforgiveness, judgement, resentment, gossip, disrespect towards authority, pride and laziness.

The atmosphere we try to maintain through the whole of Shalom's operations, whether it be in the offices or on the work trucks, including the houses, is one of love, respect, honour, kindness, patience, joy and peace. Creating and maintaining this culture is extremely important for not just the rehabilitation of the resident, but also for the successful re-integration and re-socialisation of the residents into the community. When this type of culture is your standard and you live in this environment for six to twelve months or more, it becomes normal.

COMMUNICATION SKILLS

There are many communication skills that we try to teach our residents and one of them is how to bring the truth in love, in other words, how to bring truth to somebody without causing offence. One of the ways that we do this is by approaching the person who has offended us, saying, "I don't want to be rude or disrespectful and I'm not saying what I'm about to say to hurt you or offend you in any way. I want you to know that your friendship means a lot to me and I need you to guard your heart because what I'm about to say you might take offence to. The way you responded to the instructions that I gave you before I don't feel was OK. I feel that when I try to communicate with you that you can be very arrogant. You may not feel you are, but that's how it comes across."

The person's response should be, "Thank you for telling me, I will take it on board and try my best not to come across as arrogant."

It's our job to help bring out the best in people. If we are often arrogant, we don't mean to be, but unless somebody helps us to see what we can't see, we will continue to do what we really shouldn't do.

Learning new communication skills is extremely important for a person's rehabilitation. We need to learn how to express how we feel without hurting other people and to take on constructive criticism when other people feel that we have hurt or offended them. This is just one example of how to bring the truth in love. Where we have come from when people offend us, the quickest way to fix a problem is to stick a pic in your arm, pop a pill or have a drink of alcohol which covers up the offence but doesn't deal with the root cause of the offence. Often offences are triggers for us to make stupid choices like using substances.

UNDERSTANDING THE RULES

We have many rules in Shalom and one of them is that's what's relevant for one person is relevant for every person. We don't have one rule for one person, if it's relevant for one, then it is relevant for all. All residents are given an iPod when they come into rehab which has a lot of teachings on it as well as access to radio stations.

We tell all residents that they are not to listen to any other radio station except for 98five Sonshine FM, the reason for this is that change starts here.

When no one else is around, they hear a voice in their head saying, "Listen to the football."

Another voice says, "Don't do it, you're only supposed to listen to 98five."

The first voice says, "Go on, it's okay, no one will know, it's just a football match."

The temptation is there to disobey or to obey. If you can't say no to listening to a radio station, then how are you going to say no to drugs or alcohol? We try to teach our residents to listen to the voice inside you, the one trying to teach you to be honest and truthful, to obey not disobey, because that's the voice that is going to help them change their life.

CODEPENDENCY

I have found it nearly impossible trying to help two people who are codependent (married or in a relationship) and saying that they want to change. If you take the two of them in, then when one of them starts going well and the other person is going bad, then the one that is going bad takes the one who is going well out. It's sad especially when there are children involved.

I don't know many rehab places that take couples in at the same time due to the fact they so often take each other out. The couple don't understand that when they do get taken out, it hurts a lot of people who have put in a great deal to help them change and then you lose them. I believe for couples rehab to work effectively, the two residents need to be separated for at least 12 months to focus on themselves. Generally, this doesn't happen unless one of them ends up in jail or dead.

Eventually, when they are ready for the couples' program, codependency issues may be resolved.

WHY TAKE PHONES?

Why do you take people's phones from them when entering Shalom? There are many reasons why we take phones from the new residents when entering Shalom, such as:

- Stopping drugs getting dropped off
- Giving family members a break from the abuse and hardships they have gone through
- To stop bad influences from trying to de-rail their decision to change their life
- To minimise counterproductive social media influences
- To help residents to focus on rehabilitation
- To minimise breaches of Violence Restraining Orders (VRO's)
- To minimise access to pornography and other temptations

What we do for one resident we do for all residents.

Do residents get their phones back?

Residents are entitled to get their phones back when they reach Stage 3 of the program.

WHY WE PAIR RESIDENTS UP

For the first month in the program, all residents are required to be paired up with another resident wherever they go when on external activities and events. This is extremely important for many reasons: accountability, reducing temptation to pick up smokes, steal, purchase items not allowed in the centre, medical reasons, safety or making phone calls to family who have VRO's on them. Also, all the residents are paired up for the first four weeks until they are detoxed and have learned the culture and rules of the program.

- To keep new residents accountable until they understand the basics of the program
- To minimise the temptation to pick up cigarette butts
- To reduce the risk of new residents asking the public for cigarettes and other contraband
- To lessen the temptation for them to shoplift from shops they may attend
- To stop them from ducking into a bottle shop
- To make sure they don't use a public phone to organise drugs or breach a VRO

Having someone with you for the first month can help a person to make the right choices especially when they are doing head miles. What we do for one resident we do for all residents

WHY SHAVE THE FELLA'S HEADS?

We all project an image that people perceive to fit into where we are. As soon as you look at a person, your mind unconsciously assesses the person and based on what it sees, you then set boundaries, coping mechanisms and ways to communicate. An example of this is if a fella came in your home with tattoos all over his face, you would probably look for your wallet, but if they came dressed in a suit and tie, you would probably just offer them a tea or coffee.

Because of the background of some of our fellas, they may look a bit rough around the edges when they first come in. Some have top knots, some have mohawks, and some even have mullets. Yes, that's right, mullets, god forbid. I hate mullets with a passion. A mullet belongs in the ocean and not on the back of a man's head. Here at Shalom, we have a strict ruling that if a rule is relevant for one person, then it's relevant for everyone. It's not OK to make one person do something without applying the rule to everyone, that would not be fair, so no mullets mean no long hair.

We don't allow mullets, mohawks or top knots here at Shalom. We shave all the fellas' heads, No. 2 on the top and a No. 1 on the sides.

They do it in the Army, so why not here? They have hair standards in schools, why not here? We want our fellas to project an image that says we are safe to be around, we want them to project a certain image so that people will accept them for who they are, not what they look like.

With regards to the ladies, no, we don't shave their heads.

If you have any questions on Shalom, why we do what we do or anything else for that matter, we are happy to answer as best we can, just send me an email. If for the right reasons you want to check out what we do, where we get our money from, how we are funded, what we spend it on and all that we welcome it all...

WE DON'T HAVE A WAITING LIST

We do not have a waiting list here at Shalom, but keep taking people in, that's only if we feel that they are willing to do 'whatever it takes' to change their life. That means giving up everything from mobile phones, smokes, alcohol, social media, work, etc. We will never turn a person away who is at a point where he or she will do whatever it takes to change their life. It's important to take people in then and there, when they are ready, otherwise you may have to wait years for them to come back to that point where they recognise they need help. I honestly believe that getting the person at the right time plays a pivotal role in the resident's success or failure.

IF A RESIDENT WANTS TO LEAVE

Red Hill or The Pines?

When a male resident chooses to leave Shalom, we drop them at Red Hill (Toodyay Rd) or The Pines (Gnangarra Road) which is around 4 kilometres from Shalom's main office on West Swan Road. The reason we do this is so that residents have a chance to think about the decision that they are about to make that will not just affect them, but also their loved ones who are going to be impacted by their decision.

Where we drop them off, they have a 4-kilometre walk back to Shalom or a 4-kilometre walk to the train station, generally an hour to walk with two easy to remember turns either way so that they don't get lost.

If they choose to walk to the train station, then they are saying to themselves and to us that they no longer wish to do the program. Our hope is that they would have some time to think and calm down. If they walk back to Shalom and say they are sorry and wish to continue with the program, we let them back in. Some men just choose to walk off.

If we have a male resident who we feel might be at risk and is struggling even slightly mentally, then we would either drop them at a hospital or a train station depending on the person. On some occasions, it is at the hospital if this is a person's request.

With all the ladies at Shalom, we drop them at the train station if they choose to leave. Some ladies just choose to walk off.

All residents are free to leave Shalom at any time, we have nothing here holding them.

WHAT HURTS OTHER RESIDENTS THE MOST

I believe what hurts other residents within the program the most is when a resident at Stage 3, 4 or 5 chooses to leave the program without completing it. All of the residents look up to those who are ahead of them in the program as inspirations for having gotten so far and achieved so much. They want what the other residents have achieved so it gives them motivation to try harder and follow the example of those who are ahead of them

A resident may get to Stage Four, have all their debts paid, their family back in their lives, own a car, have a job, be free from drugs and alcohol and with the approval of their families, they decide to exit the program. Many residents tell their families whatever they need to hear to get the outcome they want. Over a few phone calls or home visits, they complain about how hard the program is or how unfair it is and in reality, they are just looking for an exit plan to see if the family will cave in and support them in their wrong decision to leave the program.

This doesn't just affect the residents but all staff and volunteers who have given up their time to help them to get this far. It's not just about filling your pockets with the fruits of your hard work but also about putting back into those who are coming behind you. By Stage Four or five you should have enough strength to help those coming behind you to help them achieve what you have achieved.

When a resident does choose this path and decides to exit early, it is also the catalyst for other residents to follow in their path who are clearly not ready. In rehabilitation, you tend to make close friends with many people who are on the same journey as you which can also work out to be your downfall.

CHAPTER FIVE — PHYSICAL, EMOTIONAL & VERBAL ABUSE

With regards to abuse of any form, I believe that you really need to guard your heart and set strong, healthy boundaries to protect not just yourself, but those who you love. It's really not OK for any person to be threatened with physical, verbal or emotional abuse at all, I believe that this applies to all relationships. If you are being subjected to physical or emotional abuse, I suggest that you do not put up with it and if possible, remove yourself and your children if you have them in your care and get help from a third party to facilitate triangular communication between you and your loved one in dealing with the abuse. Triangular communication means having a third party who is not on either party's side who can act as a mediator between the two people to help bring about the best outcomes for all.

The abuser really needs to get some help in dealing with whatever it is that makes them feel the need to treat others that way, with the person who is getting abused sending a clear message to the abuser that what they are doing is simply not OK. All parties must understand that to be physically, verbally or emotionally abused or to abuse is not OK. This should be done early on and not left until there are no other options. I believe a strong verbal first warning to the abuser needs to be sent, the second time requires another verbal warning and if it continues a third time, either kick the abuser out or remove yourself from that situation.

SEPARATION

When you have separated yourself from the abuser, you need to seek professional help, then work on whatever it is that is triggering the person to be that way but work on it under different homes. I believe if any person suffers any kind of physical or emotional violence, then they must remove themselves and their children, if there are children involved, from that situation immediately.

Children usually cannot speak for themselves and must have a safe place to live free from that type of fear and abuse.

I am not saying to leave permanently but it is important that you remove yourself and those who you love to somewhere safe. Some people say that this is not possible, well, I disagree. Call the police and place a Violence Restraining Order (VRO) on them. That is a short-term order that permits the police to remove a person from a home if they are causing problems within the home and putting others at risk. VRO's are generally temporary and can be removed at any time by the department on the agreement of both parties. By getting a VRO on a person, it does not mean that you don't love them anymore or that you want them punished. It means that you are sending the offending person a clear message that what they are doing is not OK and that you don't feel safe.

WHAT'S A VRO?

A VRO 'Violence Restraining Order' can be obtained from your local police station. If you, your partner, or any person in your home are feeling unsafe in your home due to domestic abuse or violence, you can call your local police who will attend your property and ask the person involved to leave the property for not less than 72 hours.

This means that the person who has been issued this notice is not allowed within 100 metres of the property or to make contact with you in any way, shape or form. The 72-hour period gives the complainants an opportunity to attend the local courts to place a more permanent restraining order that can last for up to three years.

First hearing at Court

At the first hearing, court can make an interim VRO, a temporary order put in place while the court considers making a final VRO. The court won't make a final order until after the respondent has been told about the application. They are provided with the opportunity to come to court if they wish to fight the application and give their side of the story.

A restraining order is a court order which prohibits your abuser from doing certain things such as contacting you or attending your place of work or home address. Breaching (breaking) a restraining order is a criminal offence. The court will make the order if the judge thinks it is justified.

Anyone seeking such an order must be prepared to present some physical evidence in addition to their own written statements and testimony in court. Evidence can include photographs, text messages, police reports or medical records. The court will not entertain a simple exchange of allegations.

If your ex-lover is sending you continuous messages in the form of letters, texts, emails and via other various social media methods, they may be committing an offence constituting to harassment.

When a VRO is placed on a person, it does not give them a criminal record but send a clear message to the person that what they are doing is not OK. If a person breaches the VRO, they are generally given a strong warning the first time. The second time is a great deal more serious and is treated as such. The details surrounding the second time will weigh heavily on the judge's mind when making his decision and the third time is usually a three-month mandatory prison stay which will also come with a criminal conviction.

SHOULD YOU CUT THEM OFF?
People often ask me, "Should I cut them off?"
I know that each person knows the answer to that question, but they just need help in finding it out for themselves. This is because there is not one answer that fits every situation. No matter how much that you love someone, sometimes you must cut them off, sometimes permanently and sometimes for the short-term, depending on each case. If it is ongoing abuse

where you have tried to fix things on three or more occasions, then it's a no-brainer until you can see and experience genuine change in the abuser.

If you're caught up with a loved one in addiction, I would never believe a word that comes out of their mouth. I would expect lies, deceit, manipulation and a whole lot more. In fact, if you didn't get any of that, I would be surprised as sooner or later, when the money or assets run out, you will.

You have heard the saying, "You can lead a horse to water, but you cannot make it drink."

Well, it's the same with people. You can tell them not to use drugs and not to drink but at the end of the day, it is their choice and not yours. They are where they are because of their choices. If their choices are having a negative impact on you or others, then for a while, it is important that you set boundaries in your life so that you don't let their stuff become your stuff.

Sometimes you may even need to completely cut contact with them and tell them not to contact you until they change. Get a third party to facilitate all communication and sometimes you kick them out of your home but keep the communication going only if you feel safe and not threatened in anyway. Decisions at this point need to be made case by case.

It is not wise to continuously keep trying to push /encourage and persist in contacting them in the hope they will want to change their ways, as they will push back, and you will get taken out in the process. They KNOW what they are doing is not OK and every time you tell them they need to seek help or that they need to change, it pushes a wedge between you and them. The more that you push them, the bigger the wedge.

Alcohol, drugs and substances turn people you love the most into people you hate the most.

You tend to blame everyone else for the way that you are. To help the person you really need to know the drugs that you are dealing with as each drug will have its own set of effects. To treat the person, you need to treat and understand the drug.

They Will Say:
- You don't love me
- I blame you
- It's your fault I am this way
- I blame Mum or Dad (or anyone else for that matter)
- If my parents had not split up, I would not be this way
- I blame my upbringing
- If only you had done things better.

They will use their childhood trauma against you. They will tell you everything YOU WANT TO HEAR for them to get the outcome that THEY WANT. They will use their words like knives to pierce your heart.

DO NOT

Here are some do's and do nots. It's really important that you understand that while you may think that you are protecting your child or loved one, you may be making things worse. This is where most families get it wrong, they think they are doing the right thing but in fact, they are making it worse.

You Do Not:

- Tell lies
- Keep secrets from your loved ones
- Pay any debts on the addict's behalf
- Give them money in any form
- Pay the bills, loans, credit cards, etc.
- Pay the mortgage or rent
- Buy bags of shopping
- Pay off drug debts, no matter what the threats are
- Gossip about them to others
- Lecture them and tell them that what they are doing is wrong, by judging or criticising them
- Call rehabs trying to get them in
- Try to clean up their mess
- Send them interstate as wherever they go, they choose to go
- Drive them around.

You Can:

- Love them
- Be wise
- Be there for them in the way they NEED you to be but not in the way that they WANT you to be
- Get information on rehabs
- Take them out for a meal in a public place
- Set your clear boundaries
- Encourage them to make good choices
- Expect them to do things that may hurt you
- Expect them say things that may hurt you
- Expect them to steal from you
- Expect them to lie to you
- Expect them to blame you.

They will tell you how they need help but it's like the broken saying to the whole, "Fix me but fix me my way."

It's obvious that their way will not work because if it did, they wouldn't' be in the position they are in. Help must come in the way they need it and not in the way they want it. If they don't want it your way, then they are not ready for change.

HOOKS IN THEIR BACK

This may not sound right but you want as many hooks in your loved one's back as possible. Hooks represent pressure, unpaid bills, no food, no phone credit, unpaid rent, no fuel, drug debts, broken-down car, the threat of bankruptcy and outstanding debt letters.

The greater the pressure, the closer they will come to wanting to change. It's true.

Most families think that they are doing the right thing by doing those enabling things such as paying debts and buying food but seriously, these are the dumbest thing you can do. If it gets to that stage, well, "Houston, we have a problem."

For those who don't understand that saying, then I'll put it in another way, "The building is about to fall."

By you paying their debts, you are only delaying the inevitable. You will not only lose thousands of dollars in the process but also damage many relationships and put others at risk.

Trust me when I say that it IS going to fall.

If you try to delay it, addicts just cause a whole heap more damage in the process: anger, unforgiveness, resentment, lies, bitterness, division and more.

All these elements represent hooks and sooner or later, they will have so much pressure where they can either say, "Give me some money, pay my bills, you don't love me anymore, you are why I am like I am. I'm going to kill myself," or "I can't do it anymore, I want to change." That's the antidote for change. If you keep pulling the hooks out their backs, the longer they will keep using drugs and blaming everyone else for why they are like they are.

PLEASE DO NOT PAY ANY DEBTS

Please do not pay any debts on your loved one's behalf as the money that you spend on paying their bills just pulls the hooks out of their back, enabling them to use drugs and substances for a lot longer and in turn, their minds get worse, their health gets worse, and you are hurting a lot more people in the process. I cannot emphasise enough how important it is that you do not pay their debts.

What helps bring a person to a point of wanting to change faster is the pressures of life such as:

- Being unable to pay their bills, rent, mortgage, electricity, credit cards and other loans
- Having no food in the cupboard or fuel for their car
- May have lost their job but are not eligible for Centrelink benefits or Centrelink have cut them off
- Have nowhere to live, living out of motel rooms or couch surfing
- Having Court matters pending
- DCP may be involved.

CHAPTER SIX — TESTIMONIAL

Dear Peter,

I got married in 2013, believing the man I married to be a Godly man, and I made my vows with the full conviction that divorce was never something I would ever consider. I knew something was wrong by the end of the first week of our marriage, I didn't have the words for it then, but now I know that I married a psychologically, spiritually and emotionally abusive man. I wanted to leave within the first month (probably even earlier) after enduring hours upon hours of mental torture every weekend. I stayed because I believed that Christian's don't get divorced.

I couldn't change my husband, so I worked on myself. I tried to be more loving, more patient, more understanding. Instead of fighting back, I sat in silence and endured the verbal beatings. Instead of sticking up for myself, I tried to be more empathetic, I tried to see things from his perspective, rather than trying to have my side heard. In those moments, I would pray to God to either end my life or that he would hit me, so that I would be able to leave, because any physical pain he could cause in those moments would have hurt less than the mental pain he was inflicting. I carried no physical bruises or broken bones, but I felt beaten to a pulp inside.

When the hours and hours of lectures got too much for me and I tried to leave the room, he would block the doorway and keep me there. When I could escape and make it into another room where I could close the door, he would bash on the door or hound me to let him in. He scared me so much, I would suffer panic attacks. After hours of abuse, he would finally lose steam and then he would be terribly sweet, crying and telling me how sorry he was. He would say what an awful husband he was, and I would end up comforting him. This formed the abusive cycle I lived through for years.

I lost all sense of who I was.

I lived to please him and keep him happy. I walked on eggshells constantly. My happiness became entirely dependent upon whether or not he was happy. Anytime something was about me, like my birthday, for example, he would find a way to ruin it. He constantly berated me for having a good relationship with my family, constantly telling me I was to have less to do with them because that's what the Bible says, whilst simultaneously insisting his father spend every weekend with him fixing something in our house and insisting I entertain his mother.

I couldn't see what was happening to me and I knew I could never leave anyway. We had two children together. The psychological damage I endured while we were together was so bad that I can't even remember most of my daughter's first 18 months. I finally found the courage to leave. I wish I could adequately describe to you what it is like. I was terrified of my husband. This man who had promised to love me like Christ loves the church. My husband failed. He was unfaithful to me from the day we were married, in more ways than one. My husband broke every single vow he made.

"I didn't want to leave him."

I didn't want my children to grow up in a broken home. It broke my heart even thinking about it. But I came to realise that my children WERE growing up in a broken home. My son, who was only 4 when I left, tells me he can still remember his dad yelling at me after I had put him to bed. After I left, I sought refuge in my parents' house. I came to see very quickly a MASSIVE difference in my son's behaviour, he completely changed, he realised how angry he had been. But in the safety of my parents' home, my son didn't need to protect me, he didn't need to fear, he didn't need to be anything but the little boy that he was. He came alive and so did I.

When I left my husband, I spent the next 9 months trying to convince him of his abusive behavior. I requested the help of the elders in my church who also worked hard to try to show my husband how he was treating me was wrong. My husband refused to repent. I spent every night on my knees in prayer, seeking the Lord's Will. I had two choices: reunite with my unrepentant abusive husband, pretend our marriage was OK, and put up with his behavior, subjecting my children to the same, or leave for good, and maybe protect my children from having to watch their mother being abused daily and be abused daily themselves. I chose the latter, after much prayer and many shed tears.

I don't think I gave up on my marriage. I think my husband failed both me and my children — he gave up on us. And I think this post has the potential to shame women into accepting abusive behavior when I don't believe God would call us wives to do that. Jesus gave his life so that we could be free from bondage to sin. I don't think Jesus would now call me into bondage to be enslaved to endure abuse at the hands of an evil man who calls himself a ' Christian' (I add brackets because I don't think any man who could unrepentantly abuse his wife could possibly be saved).

Pete, I am so glad that God has worked a miracle in your marriage. I praise God for the work that you do and for the work He has called you to. I hope and pray that God would lead you to consider though, that not every marriage should be saved. Staying married for the sake of staying married at the cost of the safety and sanity of the women and children enduring abuse is not what Jesus calls us to. I pray every night for my children because I am acutely aware of the impact that growing up with divorced parents is likely to have on them. But I have no doubt that had I stayed, they would have needed just as much, if not MORE prayer for their lives because of the impact that growing up in an abusive environment would have had. I am broken-hearted that I cannot raise them in a loving home where their parents are together. I do not want to be a single parent and I must bring my shame to God every day, because I believe that shame is not from the Lord, but from Satan. I know that God rescued us from being enslaved to a man who does not bring honour to Him. Yes, the ideal is that marriage would be for life. A husband would love his wife sacrificially like Christ loves the church, and a wife would willingly submit to the loving leadership of her husband. But this does not always happen, and I strongly believe we should be protecting the women and children in such instances, NOT just focusing on fixing the marriage.

DON'T FEEL GUILTY ABOUT LEAVING

I don't believe that you should feel guilty about leaving a marriage or relationship as it does not mean it's permanent. By leaving, you are sending a clear message that what they are doing is just not OK. Some things cannot be sorted out while you live under the same roof. This is the same with addiction. If you allow a person to live under your roof while they are using and abusing drugs and substances, then what you are saying, without saying it, is that what they are doing is OK, when it is not.

They will never change while you continue to enable them, to put a roof over their heads and enable them to do what they should not be doing. If you challenge them, they will just turn on you and start to blame you for why they are like they are, when in fact, it is them. They are the ones who are making the choice to do what they are doing but you start to feel guilty because of what they say. Guard your heart from their words.

STAYING CAN BE DESTRUCTIVE

In many cases, staying can be as destructive as leaving the marriage/relationship. You must know that it is OK to know you can leave a marriage or relationship without taking on the guilt of ruining the children's lives. In most cases, you are protecting them.

If you choose to stay in a marriage putting up with any form of abuse, domestic violence, unfaithfulness or addiction, the damage that it causes you and your children will be long term and will take many years for all parties to recover. Also, by staying, you are enabling that person to do and to be something they should not. I know that many adults still suffer from childhood trauma due to their parents not protecting them when they were younger.

TOO SCARED TO SPEAK UP

So many people are too scared to speak up about what is happening in their home for fear of what others will think or that they will betray their partner or the one they love. But by keeping it in the dark, where no one knows, the problems just get bigger, so early intervention is important. By speaking up early, it can save a great deal of damage to many parties and helps in putting together a united family intervention strategy.

Darkness
- Telling lies about what's happening in your life
- Having a fear of what people may think if you speak up about the abuse
- Not speaking up due to Shame, Guilt and Fear

Lies, deceitfulness, unforgiveness, bitterness, anger, hatred, gossip, slander, being judgmental, division, destruction, manipulation, separation, they all sow discord, addiction, sickness, disease and death.

Light
- Always telling the truth, regardless of what people might think
- Being open, honest and transparent about what you are going through
- Have an accountability partner, never compromise about being open, honest, and transparent.

Love, truth, honesty, integrity, transparency, humility, being kind, caring, patient, respectful, considerate, forgiving, compassionate, empathetic, accountable, polite, these all gather us together, unifies, brings us hope, health and life.

A UNITED FAMILY INTERVENTION

By putting together a united family intervention strategy, it helps to get the immediate family on the same page. They can all come together to help the person, not in the way that that person wants it, but definitely in the way that they need it. It achieves unity, more combined wisdom and helps you to think outside the box. I know that in many cases, some family members and friends will not come on board and that's OK. They will learn, but they will learn the hard way.

How you can help everyone in coming together as one is by nominating a person in charge, someone who is emotionally strong enough to facilitate triangular communication between the two parties with clear boundaries in place, something which can be extremely effective. Examples of the best types of communication are how to respond, don't gossip, what's said in the group stays in the group. I can't emphasise enough how effective this can be if done early and how much damage this can save in the lives of all those involved, if done properly with hearts guarded.

CHAPTER SEVEN — GOSSIP CAN BE LIKE POISON

Gossip can be like poison. The more you talk behind a person's back and the more people you talk to, the faster it spreads and the more damage it does to those you love or those people within your lives. People don't need to know all the details about what is going on, it needs to be kept in a trusted circle if caught at an early stage. Boundaries need to be set and the do's and don'ts must be explained. The smaller the circle on a need-to-know basis, the better it is for all involved.

YOU MAY NOT AGREE

Please know that this book will be confronting to many people. You may not agree with everything that is written in it and that's OK. Please forgive me if I offend you in anyway as that is not my intention. Some of what you read may need further explanation. I have tried to cover as much as I can and that I know. I could cover a great deal more but what you will read is a short summary that can be explained in depth if we dig deeper, depending on the individual.

If this book brings anger, resentment or judgement up in you, then please ask yourself where that comes from? What have you been through in your life to bring those emotions up in you? Where have you been let down? These are heart issues that need to be explored.

LIVE WHAT YOU WANT YOUR CHILDREN TO BE

I don't fully understand what's happening to our society today. An example would be in the way that we bring up our children. Many of us are "Do as I say but don't do as I do," type of people. In other words, we tell our children not to do what we do ourselves, but that's not OK.

We don't have one program in Shalom. We have 150 programs because we have 150 residents from all different backgrounds. From the day a child is born, it begins to be programmed, it's programmed by the way that parents are parents, the way parents model themselves in front of the children, not just in what they say but also in what they do, in public and in private.

Our children watch the way we speak, the way we treat each other, the way we handle life's battles, they copy us. Children are also being programmed by the schools that they go to, the way the teacher teaches the kids, as well as the other kids that they hang around, the culture of people that they mix with. They are being programmed. When we live life, we all face circumstances that we do and those we don't create, which in turn gives us the outcome.

We implement patterns of behaviour, ways to communicate, set coping mechanisms as well as set boundaries in our lives to protect ourselves, to get us to where we are today. If they work for us, then they become part of who we are, we are all being programmed.

I meet hundreds of people who have come through Shalom who have said that they don't want to be like their mum or dad, yet they have turned out like them. It's not OK for a parent to say not to swear and then they themselves do so in conversations around other adults. The children hear you and see you, they may not do it around you, but they will then swear as well.

I remember a couple of years after I had started to change my life. We were sitting at the kitchen table with my wife and two kids, Peter was eleven and Rhyan was seven. I lifted my leg at the kitchen table and did a huge fart. Everyone laughed and thought that it was funny except for my wife, Amanda, who gave me a dirty look.

The next night we were sitting at the kitchen table again when young Peter lifted his leg and did a huge fart this time. He looked up at me, laughing with a look on his face as if to say, "Was that good, Dad?"

I honestly looked on in shock and left the kitchen and went into my room and cried as I thought to myself, "He is only copying me."

That was a massive wake-up call for me. If I wasn't going to fight to change the bad things about myself, then my children were going to have to fight for what I don't fight for.

I took my children aside, one on one, and sat them down to ask their forgiveness for farting at the kitchen table. I told them that what I did was wrong and that I was sorry. It's not ever OK to pass wind at the kitchen table and especially in front of their Mum, it was disrespectful. I also asked them to forgive me for the way that I was a dad, for the many things that I shouldn't do, that I needed to change and I promised them that from that day forward, I would do my best to be the best Dad that I could be. I asked them that when I do things that I shouldn't, please help me to see what I can't see so that I could do things better.

We have a responsibility to bring our children up in the way we want them to go so that they won't depart from it, not just in what we do.

There are many other examples such as swearing, fish, chips and salt words, F#@#, C#@# & S#@# words, get it? Or speaking in anger towards another person, gossip, bullying, making fun of people, stealing or driving while using phones.

If we don't fight to change us, then our children will have to fight for what we don't fight for.

I never had parents growing up. No one taught me that you are supposed to lift the toilet seat to do a pee and then put it down after you.

I had to learn to model what I wanted my children to be, to take ownership of my life, to be the best ME that I could be, the best husband, father and role model for my community. Did I get it all right? No, but I tried my best and learned to admit it when I got it wrong.

HELP US TO SEE WHAT WE CAN'T SEE

I have and will say this often, "If I am doing something wrong and I can't see it, then please help me to see what I can't see so that I can change and do it better."

I'm trying my best, help me to try better.

Many people try to speak into another person's life who are not fully informed, who haven't walked in their shoes and do not fully understand what's involved or going on. Truth should be the central point, everything that is perfect, 100 percent truth and the source of thereof. I don't believe that truth should be watered down. We are attempting to build a person's foundation for them to build the rest of their lives on.

DO YOU KNOW HOW IT FEELS?

Do you know what it feels to be all alone in a room, curled up in a ball, rocking from side to side, just wishing that you were either someone else or never born? Do you know what it feels like living your whole life asking yourself why you did not grow up normal like other people, doing normal stuff? Things like going to the one school, playing sports, having a Mum and Dad, experiencing people genuinely celebrating your birthday and Christmas with you? Do you know what it feels like to live your life trying to break free from your past, from all your mistakes and bad choices, but no matter how hard you tried, you always fell and it seemed that you could never get it right? Do you know how it feels to be locked up in a prison observation cell naked with prison officers laughing at you, while you cry in a corner with faeces running down your leg, not wanting to be alive?

Do you know how it feels to be an eight-year-old boy sleeping at a mate's house only to wake up during the night to a man giving you oral sex and molesting you? Do you know what it feels like to walk into a court at the age of nine, not knowing why you were there and seeing your Mum and Dad sitting in the court with their new partners, only for them to hand you over the government, to be made a ward of the state? Do you know what it feels like, just wanting to be a good person but trapped in a bad person's world?

Do you know what it feels like growing up watching your Mum's boyfriend constantly holding her by the hair with one hand and with the other, he was caving her face in with his fist and not being able to do anything about it? Do you know how it feels having your whole childhood stolen from you, where what should be a celebration, is in fact a bad memory filled with regret and reminders of your past? Do you know what it feels like going to school having to steal other kids' lunches because you never had your own?

Do you know what it feels like having brothers, sisters, and family who you really want to connect with but don't know how to connect due to growing up in separate homes and living separate lives?

Do you know how it feels living a bad life and then encountering God for the first time, seeing and feeling the changes He makes in your life, only to feel like you have completely failed God, let Him down and think He has cast you aside?

Everyone has a story. Everyone has been through something and all I'm doing is trying to help people, not for money but because I care. It's like my whole life, I just wanted to be a better person, but no matter how hard I tried, I always failed.

Well, now I've found the way to change not only my life but other people's lives as well. I'm not saying that I know it all or my way is the only way, there are plenty of ways, but this is mine. If you're struggling with life and your past, I'm here for you but please remember it's NOT in the way you want it, but in the way you need it.

I will give you my best, the rest is up to you.

LIVED EXPERIENCE

Did you know that 90 percent of our staff are ex-addicts or come from a background of some sort of disfunction? Ex-addicts helping addicts break free from all life-controlling issues such as Post Traumatic Stress Disorder (PTSD), anxiety, depression, pornography as well as addiction to drugs and alcohol. People with lived experience are playing a major role in changing lives and restoring families.

Within 12 months, most of our residents should have:

- Paid for their own rehabilitation
- Got themselves 100% debt free
- Have a driver's licence
- Purchased a car
- Working full-time
- Be completely off Centrelink benefits
- Have most family relationships restored
- All community service fines are paid
- Be free of drugs and other substances
- Be off all medication
- Be a non-smoker
- Have savings in the bank
- Have a whole new circle of friends

And more...

And all this costs our government and society NOTHING.

LIVED EXPERIENCE IS VALUABLE

We know that people with lived experience have a great deal to offer residents in Shalom who have made the commitment to change their lives. Sadly, I believe that they are overlooked and undervalued due to their lack of accreditation. In my view, they hold more value when it comes to our organisation in learning job-specific skill sets with lived experience and knowledge relevant to the departments that I assign them to.

I have employed many staff over the years, interviewing over 60 candidates just to get one good one and even then, they still needed to work on themselves a great deal before they could help others. This is especially so with counsellors who have the qualifications, but not the experience. Many people have become counsellors due to the stuff they went through personally growing up but still haven't dealt with these issues in their own lives. I do not believe that you can give out of your own brokenness. What's in you influences the counsel that you give as well as your perception of what you see and how you do what you do.

I have also found that many so-called qualified staff that I have employed over the years had to be retrained. What they knew and how they went about their tasks was not relevant to our working model. It has been a lot easier to employ a person with no skills or basic skills, as what they learn is completely relevant to the tasks they are undertaking, and they don't have to unlearn to relearn.

People with lived experience who have turned their lives around are a great asset to rehabilitation centres and other organisations as they are a blank canvas with so much wisdom to draw from when it comes to life experience and practical knowledge.

IT'S HARD WHEN YOU'RE NOT WANTED

Shalom House is in fact working at restoring the lives of men, women and families in our community at no cost to anyone. Everyone loves what we are doing but no one wants a rehabilitation centre in their backyard! We have purchased a 60-acre block of land for the Shalom House Hub and Men's Program, as well as a 98-acre property for Women and Children's programs. Our plan was to consolidate our operations to these two properties but we are having an extremely hard time getting this happening due to state and local government red tape.

It seems that no one wants a rehabilitation centre in their area. I know of many rehabilitation centres that are having the same problems. I have tried my best to talk to the powers that be to ask them where we can move to. They give me a suggestion, so I go there and then they tell me to take it somewhere else, so I go to somewhere else. Then they tell me to go to hell but even hell does not want us.

Rehabilitation centres do not win votes, so the politicians avoid you except during election times. The local council load you up with red tape and compliance letters, stopping you from doing what you need to and in turn, making it impossible for you to do anything at all. The government literally will not give us the time of day. We received a letter from a local resident next to where we bought, saying that "We are not welcome anywhere within the shire." Why? What has Shalom done that would cause any person, especially in this case, to not want us in that area? It's not in a built-up area, it's not in the suburbs, in fact it's in the middle of nowhere.

We have a drug epidemic on our hands, people who are suicidal, with mental health problems, we have prisons bursting at the seams and mental health wards are full. We have the safest and strictest rehabilitation centre in Australia. We are safer than having a drug user living next to you because we don't even allow our men to smoke cigarettes or swear. Not once in the history of Shalom have we ever had a police or emergency service vehicle out to attend to a problem.

Shalom House has never had one single issue with the police in the history of its operations, no police call outs, no anything; our program is that strict and well managed. I call upon the local residents to embrace rehabilitation programs like ours, to trust us and to partner with them as they work at changing lives and bringing families back together. Running a rehabilitation centre in the middle of nowhere does not work. We need residents to be around temptation, people, transport, employment and families, to have the choice to leave or to stay, to make a good choice or a bad one.

PRISON SYSTEM AND GOVERNMENT

I started at Acacia Prison in 2005 as a Volunteer Prison Chaplin three days a week. At that stage, we had around 300 plus prisoners in there, that's 300 in a few years. I was at Acacia Prison for just on five years, three days a week as a volunteer Prison Chaplin and finished at Acacia Prison in 2010 to become a full-time volunteer serving people wherever I could. When I left, they had over 700 prisoners.

I went to Acacia Prison recently and walked through the prison where they now have nearly 2100 Prisoners. I have also spoken in many of the prisons in WA over the last year and all of them are full. They are putting three men to a cell again. Most prisons have tripled in size. What they are doing and how they are handling it is wrong and needs to be reviewed. I know that Shalom's model of rehabilitation would make a massive impact on the prison system.

You can class addiction in the five categories A, B, C, D and E yet there are the three types of E's. Prison was meant for one type of E, yet they are putting them (all three E's) all in the same box.

IT'S NOT OK.

When you put a person in prison, they must project an image that people perceive to fit in with where they are, or they will get stood over and bashed, amongst other things.

You must become someone you're not so you can fit in with where you are. We need to do it differently. We need to separate the wheat from the chaff, the serious from the not serious, those people who want to change and those who don't. Otherwise, we are breeding a generation of drug addicts, criminals, men, women and children full of anger and bitterness against a system that was supposed to be set up to help people to change them and to rehabilitate them, not to institutionalise them.

I have an idea that I know in my heart that would work within the prison system but for some reason, corrective services and the government of our day just won't listen, we need to start somewhere. I'm screaming on the inside for the children who are growing up without their parents. I really hope that one day someone will listen! Families are being destroyed due to the incarceration rate, our medical service and health system is under too much pressure.

When a person does hit the wall and all of a person's bad choices catch up with them, they either end up dead, in a mental health ward, living out of motels, on the streets or in jail. Remand centres are the perfect place for the Corrective Services or the Government to sort out the wheat from the chaff, the serious from the not serious. This is where all the three E's end up eventually, all in the same place getting treated the same, when in fact, they should be identified and sorted into their categories and diverted to the help that they require. I'll give you an example, here are the three E's.

CHAPTER EIGHT — THREE TYPES OF E's

As mentioned in Chapter Two, we need to be aware of the breakdown of the E's.

E1 — Hits the brick wall and will do whatever they can to change their lives.

E2 — Swaps and illegal addiction for a legal one, prescription medication. They swap Heroin for Methadone or meth for prescription medication.

E3 — This type of E is the ones we build jails for. They are quite happy doing what they are doing and have no genuine desire to stop what they are doing and change their lives. They are also the original reason why prisons were first built to punish a person for their crimes.

E1 — Hits the brick wall and will do whatever they can to change their lives.

E1's are the perfect candidates for rehabilitation centres. They have hit the brick wall and have lost everything, family, house and finances. They show a genuine remorse for their actions and a willingness to do whatever it takes to fix what they have done and to change their lives. These are the only ones that we take into Shalom.

E2 — Swaps and illegal addiction for a legal one, prescription medication. They swap Heroin for Methadone or meth for prescription medication.

E2's are not serious about changing and are only really angry about getting caught. They like the drugs and the life that comes with it. As soon as they can they want to get more drugs, they will see the jail Psych or Doctor to get prescription drugs, Methadone, Suboxone, Largactil or antidepressants. They love the kick in the chemical and continue to ask for more or self-medicate. They just go from an illegal drug to legal ones. They are not ready for serious change and do whatever it takes to get other people's drugs while in jail.

E3 — This type of E is the ones we build jails for. They are quite happy doing what they are doing and have no genuine desire to stop what they are doing and change their lives. They are also the original reason why prisons were first built to punish a person for their crimes.

E3's are in fact the reason we build prisons for, they have no consideration for the wellbeing of others and are a danger to society. They steal, drive without a licence, molest children, rape women, murder people or even commit crimes out of greed and for personal gain. They are tax frauds, steal from the corporate world and can be violent offenders. I believe that the programs we need to put in place in jail should be relevant and structured to which E that they are.

WE ARE MAKING THINGS WORSE

It costs the Taxpayers $130,000 per year per person to keep a man or women in jail, not to mention the cost to feed his/her wife/husband and children on Centrelink payments. We are also taking out the role model from the family home. Who is the child looking up to, teaching them to become men or women? Who is leading the home? Where is Mum or Dad in those key moments of a child's life? We are destroying generations of people because of one person's stupidity. We are putting everyone in the same box. We all make stupid choices, but it's how you handle the mistakes you make that determines if you change or stay the same.

How is it that for the last 30 years, the government and the powers that be have got it so wrong? I don't want to speak badly of the government, but it has got it all wrong, the politicians are wrong.

At present, the government is spending 45 million dollars on working out how to deal with meth addiction problems but they are doing the same things as before. The definition of insanity, they say, is doing the same thing over and over again, expecting a different result. This is what our government and policy makers are doing. They are continuously doing it wrong, going on educated guesses, with minimal consultation and still expecting a different result. Rehabilitation, or in the case of Shalom House discipleship, is the way to go, not a jail sentence. I'm not saying we shouldn't jail those who deserve to be there, but for the majority of offenders, it just doesn't work.

ADDICTION IS THE COMMUNITY'S PROBLEM

I believe we all need to join together to tackle it head-on at every level. From the schoolyard to the workplace, even to the local council, as well as state and federal governments, we all have a part to play in making the changes required to bring about change, but it all starts with you and me.

Together, we can make a difference.

RELATIONSHIPS / MARRIAGE

Did you know that when a husband leaves his wife, the whole family, children and friends are massively impacted? Of the 90 percent of Shalom residents, their problems stem from childhood trauma and the separation of their parents. Marriage used to mean for better or for worse, for richer, for poorer until death do they part. It's the merging together of two hearts that over a lifetime become one.

I believe that marriage should start with a friendship that over time changes. If the friendship lasts and the couple wish to pursue the possibility of spending a lifetime together, then a commitment is made by the two parties to form a relationship whereby both parties agree not to seek another partner.

If the relationship forms over time into a lifetime commitment to each other, to put up with each other's faults and flaws that have always been there, but as a team, they commit to work together through them, as they do life together.

If the relationship is working through the ups and the downs, the trials and tribulations that a relationship brings, then by the agreement of the two parties, they decide to commit to each other in marriage, as well as to the children that they may bring into this world. This is a lifelong commitment by both parties.

I am not saying that a person should stay with a partner who is being violent or sexually unfaithful. Each case needs to be weighed on its own merits and it's not a case of one solution fits all. Violence, abuse and sexual infidelity is an instant Get Out Of Your Situation ASAP Card, but how to deal with it is a person's individual choice. Some couples separate and work through it, while for other people, the hurt and pain is just too much to bear.

It's strongly recommended that when you get married, you really need to make sure that you understand who it is that you are marrying. Do you know their weaknesses, faults and flaws? Do you understand that your decisions don't just affect you but also those you love? I feel we should not be in a hurry to have children unless we know it's going to be with our life partner. When a relationship separation happens, friends are forced to choose sides, families are forced to choose sides, children are confused and they are often forced to choose sides. Parents tell their children how they feel or what has happened and in turn, unintentionally sow seeds in the child's heart that over time, can cause a great deal of damage, unforgiveness, judgement, resentment, bitterness and confusion.

When a divorced parent meets a new partner, the child sometimes doesn't know where they fit in. If both parties bring children to the relationship, then the biological child feels the stepdad loves his or her child more than they do them. They feel like their Mum or Dad takes the side of the step-parents as a unit over their own children. This is where they want to move out to their other real Mum or Dad, but when they do move, it might not be what they expected. They feel like they don't fit in now with either Mum or Dad, as both natural parents have found new partners and now, they feel like they don't fit anywhere. They go to school one day and someone offers them a cone, a drink or a drug. They try it, they love the acceptance of the new crowd, the buzz from the substance and now they feel they have a place to fit into. The problem is this new group of friends are doing things that they know they shouldn't and the spiral continues.

GOOD INFLUENCES

We don't want new residents mixing with each other to start with, as they are new to the program and really don't know or understand the rules yet. We don't allow swearing, talking about drugs, crime or women in a sexual manner or negative way. We encourage residents to think positively about their future and what they intend to do with it. We try not to have movies, books or other literature in the houses that may trigger acts of violence, things such as pornography. We like to create a positive environment for our residents by reducing negative forms of visual media, drug use and violence as we feel that it works against the values that we are trying to teach them.

We are a holistic rehabilitation centre that doesn't discriminate due to a person's race or gender orientation and we take people from all backgrounds without discrimination. Never in Shalom's history have we ever had a police complaint or ambulance needed in the 12-plus years that we have been operating.

CENTRELINK

Centrelink's unemployment benefits system was set up by our government for people caught up in SHORT-TERM crises, NOT for people to live off forever. We encourage our residents to use it only for what it was meant for and not to abuse the privilege of receiving it, as it is taxpayer's money. Our goal for every resident is to be off Centrelink benefits within 4 to 7 months and we achieve that goal.

Most residents start two days of paid work when reaching Stage Two of our program and because they have not worked for the last three months. The first $1000 that they earn from paid work does not affect their payments as they have built up 1000 working credits with Centrelink. When they hit the four-month mark of the program, they have used up all of their working credits, therefore what they earn through paid work directly affects the amount they were receiving from Centrelink.

By the time they get to Stage Three of the program, residents are working four days per week and are no longer eligible to receive funds from Centrelink. Generally speaking, this is after seven months of being in the program. It would be more than fair to say we have most of our residents off Centrelink completely within seven months.

If a family member or friend paid the two- or four-week deposit in advance on behalf of the resident due to their lack of funds, we make sure that the first person the resident pays back is their sponsor, be it $700 or $1,400.

Shalom House does not cost the government or families anything, it's the residents that pay the funds. It's the residents who are the beneficiary of the funds and in turn, they need to pay rent and other things.

WE DON'T TAKE THEIR CENTRELINK
I charge each one of my residents $300 per week for full board and not a cent more. If a person cannot pay their rent, then we cannot have them at Shalom as we are a 100 percent self-funded organisation.

It's like a boat that has a capacity to carry 50 paying customers and they want to go from one side of the ocean to the other and get there alive. If I load the boat up with people who can't pay along with the people who have paid, then everyone sinks and that's not OK.

We are the boat, it's not our responsibility to find the funds for the passenger. If they want to get on the boat, then they will need funds from somewhere.

We are doing our bit by helping people change their lives. Shalom is affordable for everyone. No one is doing us a favour by giving them Centrelink, no one is doing us a favour by paying their intake fee, put simply, if they can't pay rent then they can't stay here as we are not able to cover their costs. When a resident enters Shalom, they must pay two weeks in advance and their funds must come from somewhere. If they are on Centrelink, it does make things easier as it gives us the assurance they can pay their rent moving forward.

IF THEY ARE NOT ON CENTRELINK

When a resident enters Shalom, they must pay four weeks' rent in advance because they are not on Centrelink. By paying four weeks of rent, this assures us that they can pay their rent while we put a great deal of our time into getting them onto Centrelink. We have many obstacles to overcome such as employment separation certificates, 100 points of ID, medical exemptions, etc. Often, we are on the phone for many hours for each person trying to sort out Centrelink issues.

WHO SHOULD PAY THE ENTRY FEE?

I believe the residents are responsible to pay their own entry fee. Many residents can't afford to pay the 2 or 4 weeks' rent so sadly, they turn to their families or friends to borrow the funds required or they don't come in. Shalom, taxpayers, government organisations should not have to pay for these people as they are where they are because of their own stupid and selfish choices. People need to be made responsible for their own choices as that's one of the ways we learn.

All Centrelink payments belong to the residents. The funds always remain 100 percent of the residents. We charge each resident $300 per week and nothing more. Each resident has a trust fund set up where it keeps track of all the residents funds and what they spend daily. We don't take all the residents Centrelink payment; we only take out of their trust the agreed rent amount which is $300 per week.

If they don't wish to pay rent, that's fine, they are more than welcome to find another place to live. All residents are more than welcome to leave at any time and when they do, the Centrelink funds are paid to the ex-resident.

Just to highlight the fact again that we do not take any resident's Centrelink payments. The government are not assisting us or doing us any favours in any way, shape or form when it comes to the Centrelink payments because they are paid to the residents and go into the resident's trust account.

We deduct $300 per week for rent which comes out of each resident's trust fund. The remainder, as well as the rent amount is always seen to be the resident's money, paid by the government for them to live.

WHAT THEIR RENT COVERS

- Rent — $300 per week
- Electricity and other utilities
- Food and basic toiletries
- Transport everywhere
- Employment Supervisor
- Employment training
- Financial assistance in getting debt free
- Medical assistance
- 100 Points of Identification
- A furnished house
- Job Training
- Mentoring every week
- myGov consolidated
- Taxation returns completed up to date
- Superannuation organised, up to date
- Family support services and mentoring
- Legal assistance (criminal and family).

All this and more for $300 per week.

WHAT THE STAFF & VOLUNTEERS RECEIVE

The satisfaction of seeing lives change. It takes a great deal of commitment by everyone involved to make Shalom House work. From the staff to the volunteers and general public, it's a team effort. Many sacrifices have been made by all involved to get Shalom to where it is today.

I don't believe it's OK for a person to willfully use drugs, have a lot of fun doing so, and when the consequences of their actions catch up with them, for them to think they can just rock up at a government or non-government organisation, expecting the taxpayer or another individual to pay for their rehabilitation. They are the ones who got themselves into their mess so they should be the ones to try to get themselves out of it and in turn, they learn in the process.

CHAPTER NINE — HOW WE GET ALL RESIDENTS DEBT FREE

Financial burden is one of the main factors in the vicious cycle of addiction. When residents enter the program, it's our Finance Department's job to paint a picture of what someone's finances look like.

Our Finance Department has dedicated staff who work tirelessly to see each and every resident break free from the chains of debt. When a resident enters Shalom House, we ensure that every resident doesn't need to carry the burden of debt along with their life-controlling issues. While the resident focuses on their program, we will communicate with creditors on their behalf, regardless of how small or big the debt is. It doesn't matter if it is a mobile phone debt or a large mortgage or tax debt.

At the two-week mark of a resident's program, we sit down and ask various questions about all possible debts they have or remember. This is highly variable as each resident's financial background is unique. Debts range from traditional financial and Line of Credit (LOC) institutions, government departments and other debts such as child support, personal loans, credit cards, mobile phones, home loans, rent, family expenses and utility services.

A comprehensive list is compiled along with a financial credit report search. This is a free credit check where companies register their debts and credit enquiries. When a debt falls into arrears or defaults, it registers on a person's credit file and also reflects if a resident is currently bankrupt. This can be quite a confronting part of a resident's program.

We will communicate with the creditors to obtain the debt information and request debts to be put on hold whilst the resident focuses on their program for a period of time.

Over the years, we have built professional relationships with many companies. We often only need to let them know we have a new resident in our program and they place the debt on hold. There is a mutual understanding between Shalom House and the companies that whilst the resident remains in our program, we are working towards achieving the end goal of settling the debt in the future.

Being stuck in addiction and paying debts on time generally don't go hand in hand; however, the Shalom House Finance Department helps residents to live within their means in the future and to stay focused on their program.

The first debt we repay is the intake fee and for some families who pay this fee, it is the first time their loved one has repaid a debt. This is a really important first step for a resident in honoring the payment of a debt.

When a resident progresses to Stage 2 of the program, this is when they are eligible to commence two days a week of paid work and start saving towards being able to pay debts back. By this stage, residents understand that debt comes before wants such as the latest joggers or nails getting done. How would a family member feel if the resident can afford to get their wants, why can't they pay their debts back? This is another step in the right direction of residents being 'others' focused and making life-long changes.

Fines Enforcement are contacted to place any fines on a pay arrangement or converted to Work Development Orders/community service. We provide a safe environment for residents to serve their community service hours.

The Finance Department works closely with the Social Services Department to ensure that residents who have payment arrangements in place for Child Support obligations if applicable, ATO tax returns are up to date and Centrelink debts are on a payment arrangement.

At the six-month mark, we have another appointment with the resident where we work together on how to achieve the end goal of being debt free.

If a resident is in severe financial hardship, they can apply for a superannuation withdrawal if they have any super or they may wish to apply for bankruptcy. We will support them in their decision. Residents can achieve becoming debt free with a combination of saving money, sacrificing of wants and strict spends per week and sometimes a super withdrawal.

Some companies will wipe debts based on the fact the resident is showing substantial change in their life and they realise how hard it can be to change your life. We appreciate the support from companies in helping the lives of men, women and families in our community.

Once enough funds are available (depending on the size of the debt), we commence debt negotiations. An example of this might be an outstanding debt of $5,000 (this amount comprised of the principal amount plus interest and any other charges) where we would make an offer of between 30-50% to settle and close the debt. This process is repeated until being debt free is achieved.

With residents who have a mortgage, if they don't already have arrangements in place, we will assist them in arranging for their home to be tenanted out or sold through a real estate agent, conditional on the situation.

For residents who have vacated a rental property, we will tell their real estate agent of the resident's circumstances and depending on the situation, we will assist the resident to terminate their lease.

The is undoubtedly an incredibly vital part of a resident's journey to life-long change. The key to how you achieve becoming debt free is determination to change in all aspects of your life, good communication, honesty and transparency.

As mentioned previously, every resident has a different set of circumstances, each case is looked at and assessed individually. We then tailor our actions to deal with each resident's debts depending on the level of debt and personal circumstances.

We have also found that companies and creditors appreciate the fact that someone is going out of their way to communicate with them, especially after countless attempts to chase debts over the years. Once these residents come into our program, it gives the creditor hope of some sort of positive outcome. We spend a great deal of time, day in, day out, liaising with people from all over, building relationships and then following through with resolutions, a win/win for both sides.

It's not an easy job to become debt free, it means a lot of hard work, determination, patience, sacrifice and a positive attitude.

WE ARE LEADING THE WAY IN HOLISTIC REHABILITATION

There is not a program like Shalom House anywhere in Australia. I know this because I was held captive to the system for 26 years. We are not wanting to boast, but let people know that we have a program that is working and could be rolled out across Australia. Our program can be adapted to suit any organisation. It can help people caught up in addiction, restore families, save millions of taxpayer funds, help people struggling with mental health issues, transform the prison system and more. Please don't knock it but come and have a look in order to make a qualified comment on what it is you see.

REHABILITATION CENTRES ARE DOING THEIR BEST

I know that all rehabilitation centres are doing their best in what they do, there is not one rehabilitation centre that is the one-stop shop for the world's problems. People need broad types of rehabilitation services as not one program suits everyone. We really must work together as a team to find out what's working and what's not, and ask ourselves, "How can we do what we do better? How can we help solve the problems our communities face?"

As you can see, the world just came together to put all their skills and knowledge together to find a solution for the COVID-19 problem. Many people have been looking for the best way to help people caught up in addiction or struggling with life-controlling issues for many years, not to mention the prisons and how we combat the growth in the system with it tripling over the last 20 years, yet we are still looking.

Well, all I'm saying is that we may have worked out a way to help a great deal of them. Please don't think I'm bragging, unless you have been out to Shalom to see for yourself, met the staff and residents, as well as looked over the program and asked the questions that you should.

Until then, you really shouldn't speak about what you are not fully informed about, and I mean that respectfully. We are doing our best, help us to see what we cannot see so that we can do what we do better.

I believe that we have gathered together what works and disregarded what does not. Please don't attack what you don't understand.

Shalom House is "Leading the way in Holistic Rehabilitation."

YOU ARE FREE TO LEAVE
"You are free to leave at any time that you feel like you have had enough."

That sounds a bit blunt and simple you might say, well, it is. No residents are ever forced to stay here, anyone can leave at any time they like. If you don't like the way we run it here, then you can simply leave, it's that simple. There are many rehabilitation centres that people can choose from. No one rehabilitation centre has the answer for everyone, and I believe that all rehabilitation centres are trying their best.

CHAPTER TEN — YOU DON'T HAVE TO BECOME A CHRISTIAN

You do not have to become a Christian when you come to Shalom. You can be a Muslim, atheist, Hindu or any religion for that matter. Please understand, we are a Christian organisation that practises the Christian faith that takes in people with all spiritual beliefs or none. Our aim is not to convert people to Christianity but rather, to help them transform their lives and to help them break free from whatever it is that they are being held captive by.

WE ARE A FAITH-BASED REHAB

I believe if the Church of God was like Hungry Jack's, it would be chockers (full), but it's not, it's made up of all these different denominations. For a person who comes from where I come from, how do you know which one is the right one? I'm not a religious person, I'm a Christian. We are unashamedly a faith-based Christian rehabilitation centre, we don't just rehabilitate Christians. We are non-denominational and residents attend services at all denominations of the Christian faith.

RELIGIOUS PERSON

A religious person to me is a person who goes around saying fish, chip and salt every second word (Fu.., C... & S...), you get my drift? They tell everyone to do what they don't do themselves: lie, gossip, look at women lustfully and go to church once a week. I can't stand religion. Have you met one of them?

A CHRISTIANESE PERSON

Well, a Christianese person is someone who goes around saying, "Hallelujah, praise the Lord, glory to God." Every second word is "God" this and "God" that, "Glory" here and "Glory" there. They set the standard of Christianity so high that I don't want to be like that and it's too hard for me. When you come from where I come from, it's a standard that, for most people, feels like it's just too hard. Now I'm not saying there is anything wrong with them. The Bible says, "I would rather you hot or cold not lukewarm, because I'll spew you out of my mouth."

I DON'T GIVE A FLYING FLOPPA

The "I don't give a flying flopper" mob say, "It's OK, I'm a good person, I'm not hurting anyone." If religion works for them, good on them, but not in my circle.

THE CHALLENGE

Well, the challenge is, if what they are trying to communicate or are saying is actually true, where a great deal of people stand right now, they are in a little bit of a pickle. I personally reckon we're not just a fart in the wind, and I reckon that when we die, there's something up there. In fact, I now know because of what I have and am still experiencing. How do we communicate what we know to be true, without pushing religion down people's throats?

I don't believe that it's OK to push what we believe upon other people, it's just NOT OK.

If we truly want to tell people what we believe, then I think we should live it. We should lead by example, in the words we speak, in the thoughts we think, in how we lead our homes and how we are with our finances, as well as how we respond when we are mistreated.

Many, many people have been hurt by religion, hurt by people who think they are doing the right thing but who are actually doing the wrong thing. When I became a Christian, I went from zero to one hundred in half a second flat. I became what you would call a God botherer. If you didn't want to hear about God, then you should have stayed away from me at that time, as I was determined to do what I could to tell everyone about what I believed. But what I was doing was wrong, yet I could not see it. I look back now and know that I did more harm than good.

I have learned more in the last ten years running Shalom House than I have in my whole life. Many men who come to us have been hurt by religion in their past and if you are one of them, "I am very, very sorry." At Shalom, we take people who are atheists, Muslim, Hindu, Buddhist, New Age as well as anyone else who has some form of faith or no faith at all. I don't care what you believe as you are always welcome here.

What is real for you is real for me. If that's what you believe, well, that's fine with me, come as you are and come with what you believe, it's OK.

What I do care about is that if you are wanting to come into Shalom to change your life, then you must be teachable. You must be willing to talk about the issues that face us including faith because here, we learn about truth, and we welcome every question as we begin the journey of truth.

I really do care about people and don't get paid at all for what I do. I'm not in this for the money, I'm in this to help people change their lives.

Do I make mistakes?

YES AND PLENTY OF THEM but I am trying my best.

If there are things that I am doing wrong, then please help me to see what I can't see, please speak into my life and help me to change. I don't want nothing from you or anyone else, all I want is for your life to change like mine did. I want honesty, integrity and transparency to be a part of your life.

One of the reasons that I write this is to let you know where I stand. I'm not pushing religion down anyone's throat, they are here by choice and can leave any time they wish. No one is holding my fellas and ladies here. I'm not selling them drugs. I'm trying to help them change their lives, I don't get anything in return and nor do I want it. If you don't like the way I do it, please don't be angry at me for wanting to make a difference. Would you rather I stop and put these fellas, ladies and families back on the streets?

Also, if you don't like how I do it, why don't you have a go doing it your way? I promise I will do what I can to support you and I really mean it. Someone has to stand up and do something. Families are being destroyed and all I'm doing is trying to stop that from happening.

Yes, I run a faith-based Christian rehabilitation centre. We don't just rehabilitate Christians even though MOST of them need it, but we are UNASHAMEDLY Christian.

Do we employ people from a no-faith background?

MY OATH WE DO.

Do we employ other people from other religions?

MY OATH WE DO, and so do most workplaces in Australia.

Acts 24:14-16
I admit that I worship the God of our fathers as a follower of the Way, which they call a sect. I believe everything that agrees with the Law and that is written in the Prophets, and I have the same hope in God as these men, that there will be a resurrection of both the righteous and the wicked. So, I strive always to keep my conscience clear before God and man.

WHY THREE CHURCH SERVICES?

The reason we go to three church services every week is because I can't stand religion, I hate it with a passion.

Please let me explain.

As I've said before, if the Church of God was like Hungry Jack's, it would be chockers (full). But it's not. It's made up of all different denominations. At least when you go to Hungry Jack's, you know what you're getting. For me, it's a Whopper double beef with cheese, extra pickle DP...!

At Shalom, I don't have one program. I have 150 programs because I have 150 residents who have all been programmed differently. If I had one program for the 150 residents, most of the program wouldn't be relevant for the person right there, because residents are all at different stages in life. All learn differently, think differently and come from different backgrounds. I don't want to push religion down the residents' throats and I don't want to be seen pushing them towards one particular denomination of the Christian faith. The reason we do go to three different church services is to show them that the body of Christ is different due to the various denominations.

FRIDAY NIGHT

On a Friday night, we might go to a Pentecostal church where they wave flags, pray in tongues and fall on the floor.

Sometimes they might dance around the room, and the services can run longer than a normal service. Having 150 residents in the program, some of my residents really like that church. They feel comfortable and it helps them to grow spiritually and interact with people who are alike in personality.

SATURDAY NIGHT

On Saturday nights, we sometimes visit a rather large church which over 5,000 people attend over the course of a weekend. It is called Riverview Church, and their motto is "The church for people who don't like church." It's a great place to bring family and friends who don't like religion or don't come from a faith background because you won't get religion pushed down your throat or some on-fire Christian sticking a flag on your head trying to lead you to Jesus because you're the new person in the church. It's a non-denominational church and I find it's a safe place for us to encourage all the family and friends of the residents to come along to spend time with their loved one. All the families who attend our Saturday night services feel comfortable and don't feel the pressure that a small church could give when it comes to religion or faith. Again, a lot of our fellas really enjoy Riverview church and some of our fellas don't.

We also conduct our Shalom House Family Nights on a Saturday. It's where the families and friends and children of the residents can come and spend time with their loved one who is in the program.

SUNDAY CHURCH

On Sundays, we go to all different churches across Perth because in our program, we have 150 residents from all different backgrounds and various suburbs. Some are from Armadale, Girrawheen, Rockingham and some from Mandurah. Other residents are even from the eastern states, from the other side of Australia.

Sometimes, we will visit the Catholic, Anglican, Protestant or Baptist churches or the Churches of Christ as well as visit many other denominations. Every Sunday, we try to attend a different denomination in a different suburb every week. The reason we do this is to show our fellas that the body of Christ worships differently. Again, I don't want to be seen to be pushing my residents towards one particular denomination as some don't fit or feel comfortable in attending certain denominations.

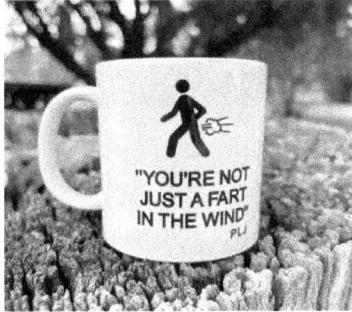

By going to all these different denominations and churches, our residents get to learn that the body of Christ is indeed differently presented. But what binds them all together is the absolutes — God the Father, God the Son, God the Spirit, salvation by faith and repentance which is outworked in actions and in truth. It also helps the residents to see that those within the church are just as screwed up as those outside of the church and that we're all on a journey to either good or bad.

I seriously do hate religion, but what if the message that religion has to proclaim is actually true? You're not just a fart in the wind. When you die, do you think that's all there is? Please, if there are things we do that you disagree with, don't shoot us down as we are trying our best to help people change their life in the best way we know how. You do things your way, I do them mine.

CHAPTER ELEVEN — WE DON'T ALWAYS GET IT RIGHT, BUT I'M TRYING

For some people, I know that we may not be doing everything right or the way that they want it. No matter what you do, you can't please everyone, but we really are trying our best. I am doing everything that I can to ensure that what we do works. I am teachable. If you can tell me how I can do what I do better, then please help me to see what I can't. So far, I have implemented everything that I believe works and disregarded everything that I felt did not. I'm always open to improvement.

YOU WILL BE PERSECUTED
I must be who people need me to be and not what they want me to be. It doesn't work for the broken person to say to the whole person, "Fix me, but fix me this way."

They are obviously broken because they are doing things their way, that is why they are broken and in the position that they are in. Families try to help them their way, but it will not work.

We all must be who people need us to be and that is hard because we love them, but love does not always come with a fluffy pillow and a warm bed. It comes with a hard decision and with facing the consequences of a person's actions. You either suffer the pain to change or the pain to stay the same, at least the pain to change disappears. I honestly say this in love.

You may not understand me, but I do what I do because I care about you. I have said this before and I will say it again, I will never be what you want me to be, but who you need me to be. When you choose to do what is right, you will suffer more than when doing what is wrong. People want what makes them feel good, not what makes them make sacrifices for their daily pleasures.

I believe people hate me because I tell them what they need to hear, not what they want to hear. Every day, I receive abuse, death threats, stalking, gossip, slander, untrue and unjustified false accusations and more. I would like to say to everyone who reads this: "I do not care if any person on the face of this planet likes me at all, I am not here to be your friend, I am here to help change lives. I will be who you need me to be and make no excuse for it."

ENABLING

One of the best ways friends and family can help and not hinder a person's rehabilitation is by working together as a team and by putting one person in charge, so to speak. It can be very confusing when a friend or family member is not on the same page as the rehabilitation centre as it works against what the resident and Shalom are trying to achieve.

I can't express enough the importance of everyone being on the same page but sadly it doesn't always happen, everyone thinks that they know best until they get burnt.

HOW TO SUPPORT

The families and the residents need to come to the realisation that what they have been doing up until the point where the resident entered the program was not working, otherwise the resident would not need to be in a rehabilitation program. It's important that both parties form a level of trust, not just in the program, but in the staff who are doing their best to help the loved one to change. Our goal is the same and that's a changed life. How we achieve that goal and how others achieve it may differ, yet we have the same goal. We have put together what we believe works and we really ask for the support of those around us in what and how we do what we do.

I find that everyone will have an opinion on how or what to do to help a person. I was once one of those people. But instead of just having an opinion, I put my opinions into action and started a rehabilitation service that has been continuously refined over time to what it is today. Many people would say it's not possible for them. Well, if that's the case, please support us in what we are doing as we have actually tried many things and kept what has worked and disregarded what has not. It's easy to criticise or say how things should be done when you're not actually the one doing the work, but when you are, you soon realise that the less you say the better. People who work in rehabilitation centres need to encourage and not be torn down or criticised as they honestly carry a heavy burden and trust me, you don't do it for money. Understanding the importance of setting boundaries is the only way forward.

NEW CIRCLE OF FRIENDS

It is important that to begin to create a new circle of friends as you will find that your old mates are not on the same page as what you are. As uncomfortable as it may be, you need to push yourself to step outside of your comfort zone to make it happen.

A good analogy might be climbing a ladder where at the top are the normal people, the geeks, the productive members of society who are free from the influence of drugs and substances. They do normal things like go on holidays with other families, play sports and go to coffee shops without being stoned or having a bottle of wine or a six-pack of bourbon in their hands. You set that as YOUR goal.

The rungs on the ladder are the stages that you have to go up to achieve that goal. It won't happen overnight but it will happen as you keep looking forward or should I say, upward. There will be people around you who you know are ahead of you who would be good influences on you who will encourage you to continue to push on and change your life.

There will also be many people from your past or people who you can relate to who will try to drag you or bring you down the ladder back into your old ways. Whatever you do, don't listen to them as you will lose the rungs that you have gained on your upward journey. Some of the people who will try to get you to do what you no longer want to do will be those who are closest to you. I had a mate who I was very close to from the age of nine, someone I knew wasn't a good influence on me nor was I on him. Whenever we got together, all we got up to was trouble. I knew in my heart that I had to cut him off but my gosh, it was hard as I loved him like a brother, but I also knew I was not strong enough for the two of us. I was at the point in my life where I really wanted to change and he was not and so I got taken out several times. I am not saying it was his fault, but if I was having a bad day, I would go to him to get drugs and he always gave them to me. He saw how hard I was trying to change and that I now had a wife and child who I was responsible for, yet he didn't hesitate to give me drugs, even though he knew what the consequences for me would be.

It does take a great deal of dedication and commitment to change your life. Breaking down your goal to change your life into manageable stages is like taking one day at a time. When you got out of bed today, you were given today as a gift to look after it the best way that you knew how, not just in the words you speak but in how you intend to change your life. You can change today because it is here and now, but you cannot change yesterday as it is gone! Even tomorrow is impossible to change because you're not there yet. If we spent all our time focusing on what we can't change about tomorrow, then we would never get what we could change done in today.

Get my drift, one day at a time, look forward and don't look back, no regrets.

OWN ACCOMMODATION

When the residents leave Shalom, most of them go back into the community and are working five days a week and only do one day per month on a voluntary roster, generally helping out on weekends with an activity. For every resident who has left Shalom at Stage Five, we will help them as a gift for completing the program by fully furnishing a house for them for free: that's all whitegoods, furniture etc.

I MAKE NO APOLOGIES

I make no apologies to any person or organisation who does not agree with how I do what I do. If you don't like it, you are free to go to another rehabilitation centre or even start your own, each one does it differently. I am not saying that I am not open to constructive criticism that will help me to improve or do what we do better. In fact, I am very open to it and I love it when I am helped to do what I do better. I know that I am doing my best with what I do and am giving it 100 percent. As I have said many times, "If I am not doing something that I should be doing, then please help me to see what I can't see so I can do what I am doing better."

Let's put what we know together so that we help change more lives and restore more families. If you don't understand why, how or what we do, please come to Shalom for a tour. I'd love to show you over the program or even work with you to start your own. You can do so by contacting me through my webpage www.peterlyndonjames.com.au

WHY THE STAGES

People ask, why the stages? Having five stages in the program is extremely important. Stages help to breakdown the overall goal or task at hand. They put short-term goals in place, dealing with the issues in a chronological way, in order to reach the long-term goal which is to change a person's life.

Over the five stages, we not only clean the resident's whole past up, but give them a solid foundation in which to build and live off for the rest of their lives.

CHAPTER TWELVE — INCIDENT PROCEDURES

How we teach all staff and volunteers the procedures in dealing with any incidents that may occur is to rate them in a category such as Red, Orange and Yellow.

RED — High priority incident unfolding / unfolded

- Aggressive or threatening behaviour
- Missing from the property or an event
- Walked off the property
- Not working with the program
- Need ambulance / police on property
- Fighting
- Smoking / drug / alcohol use.

These types of incidents are required to be up-lined straight to senior management (CEO, Families Manager or the Mentor Coordinator.

Basically, a red is any incident that may put themselves or another resident, volunteer or staff member in danger or the situation is serious enough to warrant the resident being removed from the program.

ORANGE — medium priority incident unfolding / unfolded

- Saying they want to leave
- Swearing
- Bullying
- Not participating in the program
- Being unteachable
- Disrespecting leadership.

These types of incidents are required to be up-lined straight to the House Leaders, Mentors and mid-level management, Families Manager or the Mentor Coordinator. Basically, an orange is also any incident that may upset the culture of the home / workplace / another resident / volunteer or staff members. We expect our staff to speak to the resident in order for them to work through the struggle or issues and to talk to them about how to get through it. If the resident still wants to leave, then they are more than welcome to go. It's important to always ask if they want to see a mentor and if they do, then we call the Families Department. If they do not want to see a mentor and keep walking away and not responding, then this may be elevated to a Red, which could result in their eviction from the program.

YELLOW — low priority incident unfolding / unfolded

A low priority incident would be seen to be generally poor behaviour, stirring others up, swearing, etc. You can never predict how a highly emotional individual is going to respond.

WHAT IS THE PERSON'S PROGRAM?

When we bring a resident into the program, they are signing over 100 percent responsibility to us so that we can help them change their lives. Throughout the stages of the program, levels of responsibility are handed back to the residents. Once we have done our part by fixing the problems of the past and equipping them with the tools for them to maintain what we have fixed, we also need them make the decisions that they also need to in order for them to change their lives. This is done by the residents handing over all responsibility (100%) to us in making everyday decisions on their behalf at the start of the process. They do this by personally agreeing to sign an Enduring Power Of Attorney (EPOA) document.

100% AUTHORITY SLOWLY RETURNED

Over the course of the program, the responsibility to make decisions on their own behalf is steadily returned to each resident.

Stage	% Transferred in this stage	Total % transferred back to resident
Beginning	5%	5%
One	15%	20%
Two	20%	40%
Three	25%	65%
Four	20%	85%
Five	14%	99%
Graduation	1%	100%

WE HAND PERCENTAGES OF CONTROL BACK

At the beginning, when the residents first enter the program, we would hand back 5% of control of their life to the resident. This would be at around the two-week mark of the resident's time in the program.

TOTAL RESIDENT CONTROL — 5%

ENDURING POWER OF ATTORNEY DOCUMENT

An Enduring Power of Attorney (commonly known as an EPOA) is a legal document a person can make that gives another person/s or organisation/s the legal authority to make financial and/or property decisions on their behalf.

If you make an EPOA and choose for it to start immediately, this doesn't mean you can no longer make decisions about your property and finances. But it means if you want your attorney to be able to start doing certain financial tasks on your behalf, they will have the legal authority to do so, under your guidance.

An EPOA does not give an attorney the authority to make personal and lifestyle decisions, including decisions about treatment and medical research. The authority of the attorney is limited to decisions about property and financial affairs.

The EPOA ceases the minute the resident chooses to leave our program.

STAGE ONE

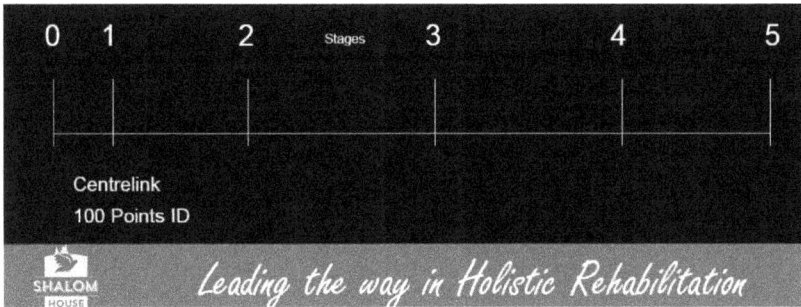

The above timeline shows five stages to the program where at each stage of the program, responsibility for a person to make their own choices are handed back to them.

Beginning: 5% control to the resident at the two-week mark.
- Responsible for making decisions on outings
- Responsible for making choices.

Stage One: 20% control back to the resident
- Identification
- Allowed to make phone calls
- Are responsible for small amounts of cash
- Reporting to Centrelink
- Cooking and cleaning
- Delegated authority on work crews.

Stage Two: 40% control back to resident

- Drive Shalom vehicles
- Leadership
- Two days of external paid work
- Computer access
- Unsupervised work and leadership
- Home Leaves.

Stage Three: 65% of control back to resident

- Allowed a phone
- Allowed a car
- Has control of all Identification
- Leadership responsibilities
- Rostered days off
- Allowed out later at night
- Working four days a week
- Paying their own bills
- Home Leaves every month.

Stage Four: 85% of control back to resident

- Working five days a week
- Takes over control of their myGov
- Looks after all their own appointments
- Medical responsibility
- Home Leaves
- Rostered days off
- Making all their own appointments
- Home Leaves every month.

Stage Five: 99% of control back to resident
- Moves out
- Own Accommodation
- Less responsibility at Shalom.

Graduation: 100%
- We can still urine test the graduate.

WE HAND OVER PERCENTAGE

At Stage One, it would be giving 15% of control back to the resident. This would be around the four-week part of the program, after we have obtained 100 points of ID and the resident's permission to cover their rent while in the program. This is normally achieved through Centrelink.

TOTAL RESIDENT CONTROL — 20%

Stage One is where you work out what a person's program is specific to the person's needs. This is done by the various departments within Shalom that each resident will sit with, usually within the first week. Starting with Resident Care, ID Services, myGov, Medical, Finances, Program Manager, Mentor/ Counsellor, Doctor, Psychiatrist and Employment or Works Coordinator.

- You identify any heart issues they may have
- Work out their family structure
- Identify the people they may have hurt or have un-forgiveness towards
- Assess their financial situation
- Identify what general issues they may have that will distract them from their rehabilitation
- Are there any medical issues that need to be dealt with?
- Are there any mental health issues?
- Current issues needed to be dealt with that will limit their focus in life and the program, motor driver's licence (MDL), etc.
- What do they want to do with their life, work, etc.

CHAPTER THIRTEEN — LIFE PROGRAM

We don't have one program in Shalom that works for everyone. If we have 100 residents then we have one hundred programs, if we have 150 residents, then we naturally have one hundred and fifty programs, as every resident has their own unique program.

The picture on the following page helps you to identify a person's program taking into account the five main areas: family structure, heart issues, general issues, financial issues as well as what do they want to do with their life direction.

After you have gathered this information from the resident, it's now a matter of breaking it down and working through it. The Popplet image is a holistic overall timeline/picture of a person's life, made up by five main headings. This first one identifies the family structure and a little bit about what's been going on.

FAMILY	PERSONAL DEBT	GENERAL	RESIDENT	DIRECTION IN LIFE
Mum	Home Loan	Rental House	Psychiatrist	Carpenter
Dad	Intake Fee	No MDL	Psychologist	Barista
Brothers	Credit Card	Pawn Broker	Finances	Painter
Sisters	Phone Contract	Centrelink	Doctor	Plumber
Uncles	Credit File	Car in Impound	Counsellor	Boilermaker
Aunties	Personal Debt	Superannuation	Home	Hospitality
Grandparents	Car Loan	Taxation	Employer	Administration
Wife	Child Support	100 Points of ID	Job Network	Accounts
Children			Mentor	Labourer
Extended Family			Courts	Plant Operator
			DCP	Rigger / Dogman

FACILITATOR OF HOLISTIC REHABILITATION

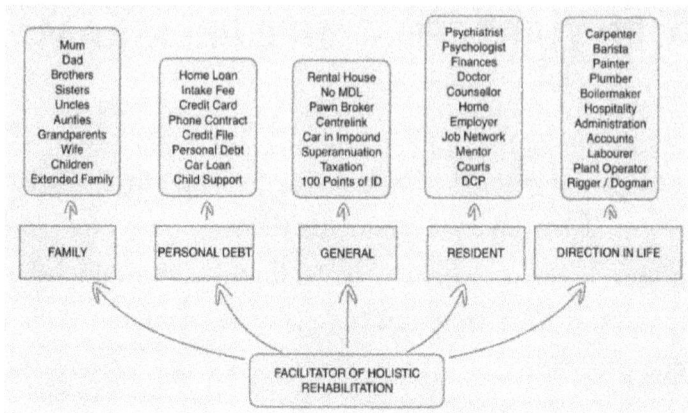

The picture on this page helps you to identify a person's program taking into account the five main areas: family structure, heart issues, general issues, financial issues, as well as what do they want to do with their life direction.

SISTER 39 · HUSBAND · 3 CHILDREN
AUNTY · 3 CHILDREN · SISTER 40 · HUSBAND
WIFE · BROTHER 41 · AUNTY
AUNTY · NAN · UNCLE
UNCLE · MUM · POP · DAD · POP · NAN
POP

PAUL 37

SON 2 2 YEARS OLD · DAUGHTER 1 4 YEARS OLD · WIFE 2 2 CHILDREN · WIFE 1 3 CHILDREN · DAUGHTER 1 13 YEARS OLD · SON 2 9 YEARS OLD

NEW PARTNER · SON 3 7 YEARS OLD

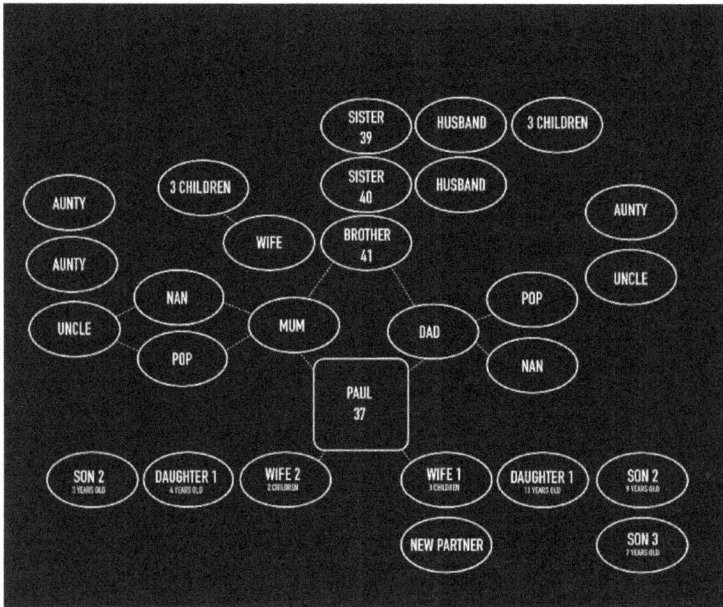

In this case, we have a 37-year-old male named Paul. He is the youngest of four siblings with two older sisters and an older brother. The siblings are all married with children except the second oldest sister who has no children. Paul's Mum and Dad are still together. On his Mum's side, Paul's Nan and Pop are still alive. They have four children altogether, two aunties and one uncle to Paul, where his Mum is the youngest of the four.

On Paul's Dad's side, his Nan and Pop are both living. They have three children, where Paul's Dad is the oldest, with Paul having one uncle and one aunty.

Paul has been married twice, with three children to his first wife and two children to his second wife. Paul met his first wife when he was 16. They were childhood sweethearts who fell in love, went to lots of parties, used drugs and alcohol recreationally and had a lot of fun doing so. One day, his first wife became pregnant, so she stopped using drugs, but he kept going. She wanted him to stop and start focusing on his family, but he saw no harm in it as he was having fun with his mates. They end up having two more children. By then, Paul had finished his apprenticeship and was working as a tradesman. They had gotten married, bought a house and a car and were living a semi-normal life.

They always argued about Paul spending money on beer and drugs. Again, he could not see the harm in his alcohol and drug use, saying that he had worked all week and that he was entitled to it. No matter how hard they tried, Paul and his first wife could never get ahead financially which caused lots of problems in their marriage. Over many years, they had many heated arguments. His wife said she had had enough of it several times.

On many occasions, Paul was kicked out of his family home, so he went to one of his other relatives' houses: his parents, grandparents or one of his siblings.

The sad thing was that everything that happened at his family home also happened at his other relatives' homes. The lies, the deceit, the abuse, coming home at all hours or sometimes not at all. The family had had enough, as he had gone from one place to the other. One day, his wife decides to have another go at the marriage. Paul told her everything she wanted to hear to get her back, so she let him move back in, and it happened all over again.

His first wife finally kicked him out and said, "Don't come back, Paul, until you have done a rehabilitation program and then I might look at taking you back."

Paul's wife loved him, but she just could not do it anymore. So Paul moved out back to his Mum and Dad's place. All the family was telling them they were making a mistake by letting Paul back in, but his parents' reply was that they couldn't leave him on the streets.

Everyone was angry, not just at Paul but also with his parents, for giving him a place to stay. He had used them, stolen from them, borrowed money and never paid it back. Why does he need rehab when other people will give him a place to stay, feed him and his habit?

Paul hit the drugs even harder than before, feeling sorry for himself, telling everyone that his wife was to blame as it justified him doing what he knew he should not do. One night, he went to a party with a few of his mates and met a girl ten years younger than he was at the time. He feels the 'fluffies' for her. You know, that emotion that comes on you when you first start to fall in love.

They begin to date and no longer is his first wife the focus. Paul finds something new, something exciting and wants it like a drug. His first wife hears about him having an affair, custody battles for the children begin and lawyers are now involved. Meanwhile, he is cleaning his act up for his newfound love, hiding all his faults and flaws, to win her over. He spends a lot of time telling his new girlfriend what she needs to hear to get what he wants, his new girlfriend takes his side while only knowing his side, not knowing all the other stuff.

Time goes by and his new girlfriend falls pregnant. They decide to get married, so he files for a divorce from his first wife, and they marry.

After their first child is born, Paul's second wife starts to see patterns of behaviour in him that she has never seen before, or did not want to see, as she was pregnant and did not want to feel the shame from her family and friends.

A couple of years later, they have their second child. Life has not been great in those four years. Every now and again, Paul goes out all night, comes home very late. There is never any money and funds keep going missing from their accounts. Everything that happened with his first wife is now happening to the second one.

She has asked him many times what he has been up to but all he ever does is attack and defend. Paul is full of lies and she knows it, but she just can't prove it. It causes anger, bitterness, resentment and a lack of self-worth about herself. She can feel herself changing into a person she does not want to be.

Paul's second wife feels that she needs to move out, but she worries about what people will think of her. What will her parents think? She never thought that she would be a single mum with two kids, so she tries to hang on. She hears all the stories from friends about his abuse of drugs, stories of him with other women. She tries to cast them aside, but they are eating her up like a cancer in her bones.

That is, until one day when Paul disappears for two days, his phone is off, and funds have been drawn from their account. She just sits at home crying, she loves him, but she can't do it anymore.

When Paul eventually comes home, his wife confronts him yet again, but all she gets is lies. By accident, she finds drugs in his pants as well as a condom. She has had enough, so she finally kicks him out. He gets verbally violent, so she rings the police and puts a VRO (Violence Restraining Order) on him and tells him to go sort his life out.

This second wife of Paul has had enough and has no plans to put up with it anymore.

Paul rings his parents, asking to stay there. They tell him that he can't, because of the pressure coming from other family members and also due to what they have been through in the past with him. He asks his brothers and sister, and they also tell him "No," and tell him that he needs to go to rehab.

Paul has no intention of going to rehab and finds a mate who will put a roof over his head. Everything that happened with his wife and family then happens with his mates. His mate ends up having enough of Paul and kicks him out after a fight, and now Paul has nowhere to go. His mind goes through all the options, trying to find the easy one. His family won't have him, his second wife won't have him, and all his mates have shut the door on him. One night on the way back to his motel room, three men from the pub mug him and take all his money. He is in a bad way.

He rings his wife crying, telling her what happened and that he loves her. Would she please take him back? Her response is "No, you need to go to rehab," then she texts him a list of rehabilitation centres to choose from. Then she hangs up. He does the same with his mum, his grandparents, brother and sister and have all responded the same.

They say, "You need to go to rehab," then text him a list of rehabilitation centres to choose from, and then hang up on him.

He has no idea that all the family had come together to put an intervention plan together to help him.

Not in the way Paul WANTS it, but in the way he NEEDS it.

He is at the bottom of the bottom, with nowhere else to turn. In his mind, he says, "I need to go to rehab," and he finally makes the call.
Not because he HAS to, but because he WANTS to.

A seed has been planted in his heart: "I can't do it anymore; I want to change."

Does he listen to the Darkness or the Light?

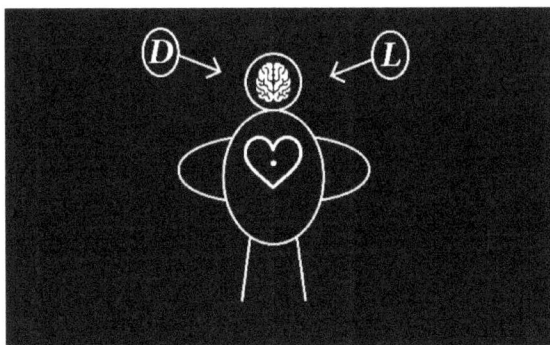

I know how to water that seed and make it grow; this is where change starts.

HEART ISSUES
I believe that your heart acts like a hard drive, a bit like a computer. Out of the heart flows the issues of life, or out of the heart flows the consequences of life. So as a man, a woman or a child thinks in their heart, so are they. I truly believe that what's in your heart influences what you believe, the way you think about yourself and the way you treat others.

As well, what's in your heart influences the boundaries that you place or set in your life, depending on what it is in your life that you have been through, both the good and the bad. If the boundaries that you implement or put in place in your life work for you, then they form a part of who YOU ARE.

Not everything you implement is good, but if it works for you then you believe that it's OK. We should always guard our hearts to let only the good in. The heart is the wellspring of life. It's where we draw wisdom from that helps us to make decisions for living everyday life.

When looking at a person who has reached rock bottom in their life, you need to find out what the root causes are. Why are they the way they are? Where did all this mess start? What have they been through that has made them this way? What is the root cause of their problems? What lies have they believed that have become their truth?

I would start with their childhood. Have they experienced any trauma of any kind growing up? Have they been sexually abused or been caught up in pornography? Have they experienced a separation of any kind? Have they moved from another country and feel like they don't fit in? Has there been a death in the family? Were they bullied at any stage? Are they struggling with fear or anxiety from something they have been through or from a confrontation with someone?

I would also look at what they are feeling personally about what they are going through, as well as how they feel about themselves. Do they hold unforgiveness, bitterness, resentment or low self-esteem in their heart? Are they carrying guilt, fear or abandonment? These are all heart issues that need to be addressed. They are the root causes of what they are struggling with, the seed that has made a tree of bad things happen in their life, but they don't know it.

They live life, going through the same crap over and over again, trying to fix the bad fruit on the tree, only for it to grow back again and again and again.

Unless you take the axe to the root and remove the seed, you will always be fighting to remove bad fruit.

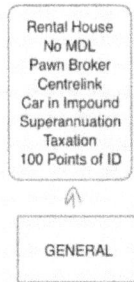

```
┌─────────────────┐
│  Rental House   │
│     No MDL      │
│   Pawn Broker   │
│    Centrelink   │
│  Car in Impound │
│  Superannuation │
│     Taxation    │
│ 100 Points of ID│
└─────────────────┘
         ↑
┌─────────────────┐
│                 │
│     GENERAL     │
│                 │
└─────────────────┘
```

GENERAL ISSUES

When a resident comes into the program, we need to do whatever it takes to help them to focus on the program and in changing their lives. We sit with every resident to find out what is on their minds and what's troubling them.

Here is a list of some examples of what comes up.

- They have a rental property that needs cleaning up
- They have a car in the impound yard
- There is stuff at the Pawn Brokers that belongs to other family members
- They owe money to a drug dealer
- They have stolen goods in their possession
- They have court proceedings coming up
- There is a bench warrant for their arrest
- They don't have any extra clothing other than what they are wearing
- They don't have the intake fee.

Depending on what comes up will influence what we do at this stage. When we have identified what may distract them from committing to the program, we do whatever we can to bring peace to their minds. An example would be if this resident had a rental property that needed cleaning up and the keys handed back. Shalom would send a team out to the property to clean it up and hand the keys back to the property manager. If there were goods at a Pawn Broker that they had stolen from a family member and it was about to expire, I would work with the resident ANYWAY to make sure that they didn't lose the property. This is an example how we work at fixing the resident's immediate issues, with the not-so-important issues being dealt with later on as they progress through the program.

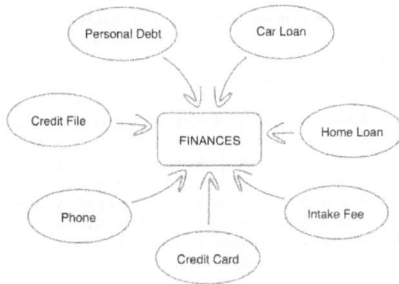

FINANCIAL ISSUES

Most people come in and their lives are a mess. After sitting with them and identifying what issues they may have, we also apply for a copy of their credit file that shows us where all the registered bad debt is listed and who it's listed to. Every resident in Shalom will graduate 100 percent debt free with all their financial history repaired and up to date.

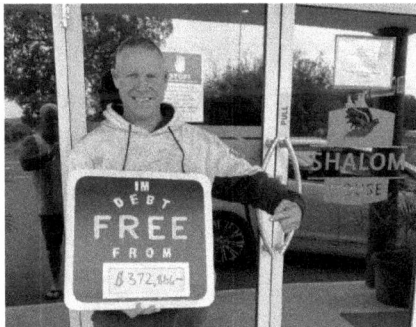

After getting the resident to sign an EPOA document, we first obtain 100 points of identification for them. Then we create a myGov account in the resident's name. Upon the creation of their myGov account, we then streamline all government departments under the umbrella of MyGov (Services Australia (formerly the Department of Human Services), such as:

- Australian Taxation Office (includes superannuation)
- Centrelink (completing the process for JobSeeker, Age and Disability Support Pensions) with myGov online (for residents to regularly report their job search activities and other mutual obligations to satisfy their JobSeeker requirements)
- Child Support
- Medicare (for vaccination proof necessary for jobs).

There are also several different types of pensions that can be processed through the Department of Veterans' Affairs (DVA) for former ADF men, women and disabled veterans. This supports veterans if they are unable to continue working after leaving the ADF.

When the essential online process is completed, we arrange for our accountant to bring all the resident's taxation returns up to date as well as locating their superannuation. We consolidate all super accounts into one. We work with Child Support to sort out the correct amount owed and put a payment plan in place depending on the resident's cashflow.

With regards to outstanding bills such as credit cards, home loans and vehicle loans, we contact the agency concerned and inform them of the resident's financial situation. We request a three-month freeze on the debt until we can come up with a payout figure or payment plan.

Each resident's affairs are different and each action that we take strongly takes into consideration how they are going within the program. This includes what stage they are at as well as how long they have been at Shalom.

No person graduates Shalom House without having all their financial debt cleared.

Cleaning up the mess

- They don't have a myGovID
- They don't have 100 points of ID
- They don't have a valid driver's licence, Medicare card, or Birth Certificate
- They have never lodged their tax
- They have superannuation accounts all over the place
- They owe thousands of dollars in child support
- They are not currently on any Centrelink benefits
- They have a car loan, a house loan or credit cards
- They are in default for all their loans and bills, electricity, phone, water, rates etc.

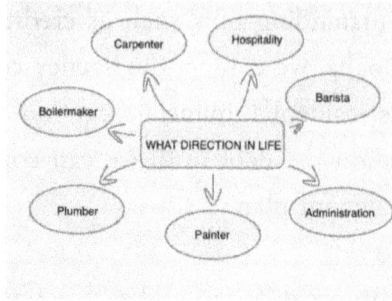

DIRECTION FOR THEIR LIFE

As I have mentioned many times, we don't have one program, we have 150 programs. We have 150 residents who come from all different backgrounds, they think differently, they learn differently, and each person has a different set of skills and abilities that will assist them in their direction in life.

In other words, what do they want to do with their life? Do they want to work in administration, hospitality, in the mines, be a boilermaker, rigger, plumber or a mechanic?

IDENTIFY LIFE DIRECTION

It's really important to find out what direction a person wants to go with their life in regard to employment and/or training. At the two-month mark of the program, all our residents will complete a National Construction Industry White Card course which gets them ready for external employers. We have many external employers from all trades and industries: plumbing, manufacturing, manual handling, transport, fabrication, labouring, FIFO/mining and machine operators as well as many other types of work.

After sitting with our employment person, we try to identify what direction the resident wants to go in, so that at the three-month mark of the program, we can pair them up with an employer who is on the same page as us.

Getting a person employment is not just about giving them a job, it's about making sure that we get them work with an employer who will actively participate in their employment while further developing their skills in a satisfying career. This is an employer who will go out of their way to make sure that the resident isn't teamed up with somebody in the workplace who is using drugs or substances, but rather, team them up with somebody who's going to be a good influence in our resident's work life.

Shalom House would like each employer to take an active role in our residents' lives within their workplaces, to partner with us to bring about the best outcome for every resident's progress for the future. We can tell by our resident's communication with the employer if they are putting into place what it is that we've taught them within the rehab. We can also tell if the place of employment is having a positive or negative effect on a resident by their attitude when they are back in the houses.

Work for every resident starts off at two days per week, then over time, it becomes three days then progresses to four days a week. By then, the resident should be at Stage Three or Four in the program.

This process continues where eventually the employer takes them on full time. It's really important that we can get employers to partner with us in changing lives. This only happens if employers take an active part in our residents' lives.

STAGE TWO

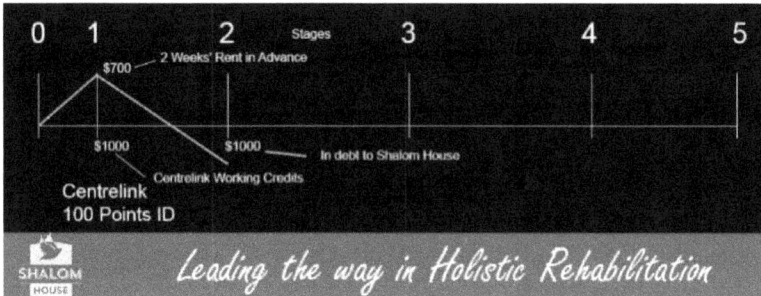

Stages: 0 1 2 3 4 5

$700 — 2 Weeks' Rent in Advance

$1000 $1000 — In debt to Shalom House

Centrelink Working Credits

Centrelink
100 Points ID

SHALOM HOUSE — *Leading the way in Holistic Rehabilitation*

At Stage Two, it would be another 20% of control given back to the resident. This would be at around the three-month mark of the program.

TOTAL RESIDENT CONTROL — 40%

When the client has been with us for approximately 8 weeks, the Directions Department sit with each individual to map out a plan for their future. No matter what the resident would like to do with their life, we do our best to come alongside them to make it happen.

Whether it's starting a business, going to TAFE, taking up an apprenticeship or completing a trade that was never finished, we believe it is possible.

Beginning paid work depends on what a resident decides they want to do in the future. We endeavour to have our residents started in their chosen field. After 12 weeks, depending on their progress and attitude, we give them the opportunity to start two days a week paid work with an employer who is on the same page as the rehabilitation centre.

Being on the same page means going out of their way to provide a safe working environment for our resident, making sure that our resident isn't teamed up with a person struggling with addiction or with other issues that may rub off, but rather, someone who will be a positive influence on their life.

The income the resident receives while working is used to help them move forward financially in their life. We begin to facilitate paying out their unpaid fines and debts that they may have accumulated. We also help them get their driver's licence or to buy a car, if possible.

We find this gradual progression back into the workforce helps us monitor whether they are putting into practice what we are teaching them at Shalom House. If there is any reason for concern, we taper it back to where we feel they need to be. This balance provides us with an opportunity to see if they are maintaining their progress, by making the right decisions and monitoring the way they behave.

A REGULAR ROUTINE

One hundred percent of the income that the residents earn during paid work goes to the resident which is placed in each resident's personal trust fund. The funds that the residents earn in paid work are used to help all the residents' get debt free, to purchase a car and pay for expenses such as necessary medical and dental fees, for example. If they have no bills or expenses, then they start accumulating funds. The two days a week paid work with their employer, who is on the same page of the rehab, is extremely important, as we begin to work out handing responsibilities and choices back to the residents. They should have been paired up with an employer where they can learn the skills relevant to their workplace direction and hopefully, they will be carrying out tasks relevant to their future direction in life. The other three days a week where they are not working outside of Shalom, residents are working on various work trucks and within Shalom to develop their workplace training skills. They could be studying to upskill themselves or complete unfinished education, such as Years 10 to 12.

Unsupervised freedom from Shalom in the workplace is extremely important, not just for reintegration back into the community, but also re-socialisation with those within the workplace. Meeting new work colleagues and building relationships outside the 'Shalom bubble' help to build up their support base and social network. When you come from a culture of people using drugs and substances, you do a lot of things that you shouldn't. So, breaking off unhealthy ties and creating new ones is pivotal in moving forward.

MENTORING

All residents are assigned a mentor to catch up with at least a couple of times every week, to see how they are going as they move through the various stages of the program. Things will be discussed such as how they are going with paid work, what temptations they faced and how they handled them. Another important aspect of these talks is centred on how they are handling the balance between paid work and the program as well as regular discussions about their families.

These specific mentoring sessions often bring necessary personal issues to the surface for the resident.

SOCIAL EVENTS

Shalom House attends many community-based social events in a voluntary capacity. One of the things that we try to make a difference in our community by volunteering, whether it be at the go-kart festival, local community events, emergency fire cleanups or even the local speedway performing traffic management duties. We also attend many fun runs, charity walks, awareness days and high teas.

HOME LEAVE

Home Leave is considered a privilege, not a right nor an expectation. A resident's first Home Leave is allowed after the resident has been in the program for around three months. They are allowed to go home over a weekend, from Friday to Sunday, to an approved person's house, generally a trusted family member.

The second Home Leave can happen two months after the first one occurs, generally around the five-month mark of their program and the third Home Leave is allowed monthly after that for the duration of their stay in the program. These Home Leaves can be cancelled at any time due to any resident's poor behaviour and choices. Home Leaves are also a way for the resident to put into practice what they've learned within Shalom House at home in an unsupervised environment. In most cases, the Shalom resident now displays a much higher level of character while on Home Leave, creating some engaging discussion with their mentor afterwards.

LEARNING FROM THOSE WHO ARE AHEAD

When I was first started Shalom House, we grew quickly. I had to place Stage One residents in one House and the Stage Twos in another. Then when my numbers grew again, I had to develop the program up to Stage Three and had to get a bigger property where I could put all the residents from all Stages into one property. I had no idea of the positive effects that this created for the residents concerned. By putting the Stage Ones, Twos and Threes together, the program gathered momentum. The Stage Ones saw what the Stage Twos and Threes had already achieved, and they wanted it all: the freedom, family visits and the trust to be unsupervised. I also noticed that the Stage Twos and Threes had put a lot of effort in coming alongside all the new fellas in Stage One. By utilising the Stage Threes as an example, we are putting hope back into the Twos and Ones, while they are looking forward and learning from those who are ahead of them in the program.

INCREASED PAID WORK

Throughout the Stage Two part of the program, the residents' paid work increases again, depending on the attitude in the workplace and at home. We increase the paid work from two days to three days then to four days full-time paid work again.

One hundred percent of the income that the residents earn during paid work belongs to the resident and goes into their personal trust account. The funds are then used to move the residents forward in life with regards to finances, such as purchasing a car and getting ready for Stage Three where they will be allowed a phone and more freedom.

STAGE THREE

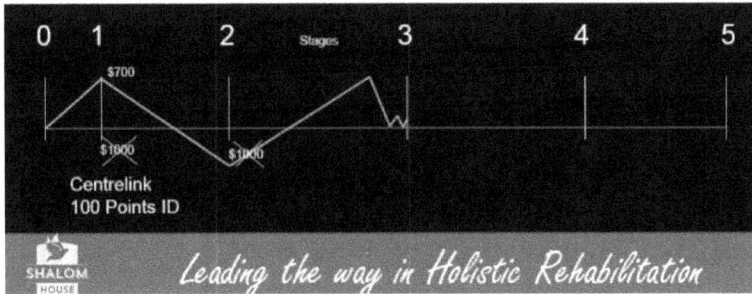

Upward movements of the line is paid work and downward movements are debt repayments.

WE HAND OVER PERCENTAGE

At Stage Three, we hand another 25% control of their life back to the resident. This would be around the eight-month mark of the program.

TOTAL RESIDENT CONTROL — 65%

Stage Three sees the resident increase the amount of paid work externally and they continue to plug in with residents who are in the earlier stages of the program.

At this point, we allow the resident to purchase a mobile phone, as well as the freedom to come and go from the Shalom House properties with an 8:30 pm curfew from Monday to Sunday. This gives the resident a greater sense of freedom and responsibility whilst keeping them accountable to the leadership at Shalom.

Steadily increasing freedom creates windows away from the 'Shalom bubble,' to test the resident's resilience. They tend to grow in their independence whilst knowing there are people to fall back on and continue to receive guidance for the issues that arise for them.

It's the Stage Three's job to make sure they put back into the residents coming behind them while learning from the Stage Fours and Fives in front of them.

It's all about discipleship.

BENEFITS

- Unsupervised freedom in the community
- Mobile phone
- Car
- Privileges of a Stage Three
- Rostered days off
- Putting back into those who are coming behind
- Drives to work alone.

CHAPTER FOURTEEN — SHOPPING

Every Sunday, all the residents are taken down to the shops so that they can do their weekly spends. No resident under Stage Three is allowed more than $50 on their person at any one time. Residents from Stages Three to Five are allowed up to $100, but not any more than that. It's the Stage Three residents who also supervise the other residents at the shops to make sure they don't do anything they shouldn't. All residents are paired with another resident on outings such as this.

They are not allowed to purchase any form of energy drink, high-level caffeine, protein powders or anything else for that matter that they may abuse or may give them a kick, if you know what I mean. If they are urine tested or breathalysed and it comes back positive, we explain to them that we will not be accepting any plea other than guilty. It is their job to make sure that they don't purchase or consume stuff from the shops that will show up as positive on drug or alcohol tests.

LEADERSHIP OPPORTUNITIES
All residents will be placed in various leadership positions to teach them not just how to lead, but how to also make good choices under pressure. This helps in not only teaching them wisdom, but also responsibility and the gift to be able to think outside the box.

Many people don't look at the bigger picture.

If you tell them to move a pile of dirt, then they will move the dirt without actually thinking where they should place it. So, they move it from one place to another, fixing one problem while just creating another. We try to teach the residents to begin with the end in mind, by asking them to picture what they want the end product to look like.

We tell them to take into consideration the pile of dirt and ask themselves how they can move the dirt to create the end product, which would be no more piles of dirt at all. Depending on the job, the right move would be to put small piles of dirt all over the place and spread it out. This should give you the end result, but not everyone would think that way.

All residents will be in leadership at one stage or another, as it helps them to grow in many areas. No matter the age of a resident, he or she will be leading somewhere along the line. When you have an 18-year-old leading ten ladies or men, it is humbling, and you do learn a great deal.

This is an example of our leadership structure:

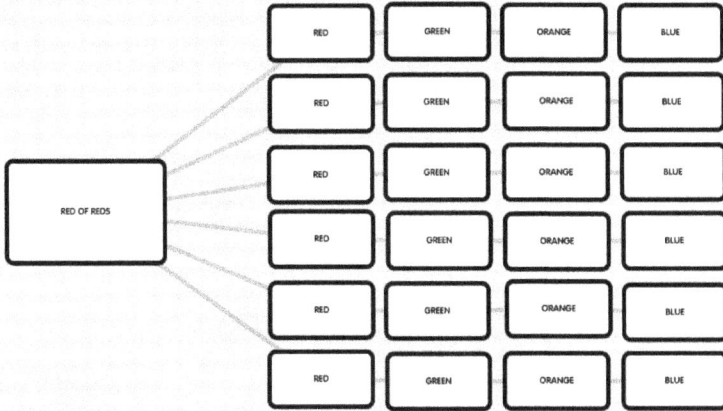

RED OF REDS	RED	GREEN	ORANGE	BLUE
	RED	GREEN	ORANGE	BLUE
	RED	GREEN	ORANGE	BLUE
	RED	GREEN	ORANGE	BLUE
	RED	GREEN	ORANGE	BLUE
	RED	GREEN	ORANGE	BLUE

- Red of Reds — he or she is in charge of all residents within a property which may have multiple Houses

- Reds — Leaders of each House

- Greens — 1ic (first in charge) of each House

- Oranges — 2ic (second in charge) of each House

- Blues — are all other residents.

We have the Red of Reds who teaches the other Reds how to teach the Greens. The Greens then teach the Oranges, and the Oranges teach the Blues who are the residents. Every House will have a Red in charge who teaches the Green who will then teach the Orange, the actual person running the House. If residents have any concerns, they must first approach the Orange (2ic). The Red Leader checks that all leaders are being giving the correct instructions on how to run the house, overseeing the entire process.

Most of our properties have two or three houses on them, so we would have a Red, Green and Orange at each House. The Red of Reds oversees all Reds across all properties. His or her job is to catch up with all the Reds at least twice a week, making sure that they are being properly trained for their leadership roles. They ensure the Reds are sticking to the boundaries of their roles and with regard to the authority that they have in their particular positions.

The Red of Reds must also put the rosters together, so that all the Stages know what days they are on roster for week/weekend events and outings.

We move all residents around across all houses every six weeks to help them grow. We ask every resident to pack up their gear and clean their rooms to a very high standard. All the rooms in all houses hold a minimum of two people per room. We move all residents around to different rooms and in many cases, to different properties. We look for people who do not get along with each other and we place them in the same room. We try to bring out the worst in the residents so that we can bring out the best in them, and it works.

It also helps having many houses and properties because it assists us in separating those with strong personalities, so that they are not bad influences on others. We have a zero tolerance to violence in the whole of Shalom. That means both physically and verbally.

'Roosters' are not allowed in Shalom. We are all fluffy chickens who must get along. If anyone tries to be a rooster, they are kicked out of the program as it is not tolerated. The leaders have a large job on their hands. They are not only to teach what they have learned, but they are also responsible for the smooth running of the houses, maintaining a strong and respectful culture within the home, free from offence.

CHORES IN THE HOUSES

- Cook meals
- Wash dishes
- Clean corporate linen
- Make beds
- Wake up times
- Clean floors, windows and walls
- No shoes in the houses
- Put shopping away
- Clean bins, BBQ
- Personal hygiene.

We have many people who come to rehabilitation who have never cooked or cleaned. They are used to sleeping until whatever time they choose. Some have a high standard of living, and some have a low standard. We have a medium standard that is required by all residents, and it is everyone's job to make sure that this standard is maintained.

Those with a high standard are brought down to a medium standard, those with a low standard are brought up to a medium standard, if you get what I mean. Our medium standard is still a very high standard that I believe all of society has, as it's standard normal.

Rehabilitation is not just getting people off drugs and substances, it's about the whole of a person's life, inside and out. How they live, what they eat, what they say, how they treat others, how they respond to others, what time they wake up, how to get ready for work, how to pack lunches, how to clean, how to respect others within the home or workplace and a whole lot more.

STAGE FOUR

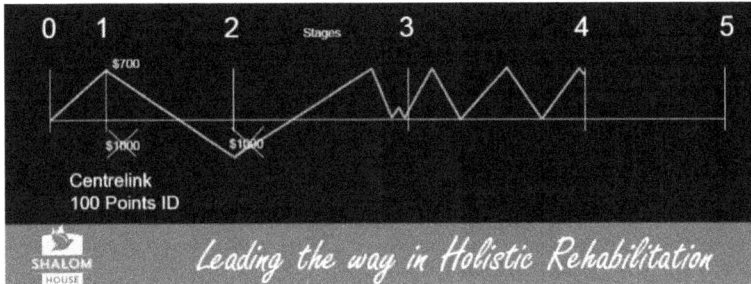

| 0 | 1 | | 2 | Stages | 3 | | 4 | | 5 |

$700

$1000 $1000

Centrelink
100 Points ID

SHALOM
HOUSE   *Leading the way in Holistic Rehabilitation*

WE HAND OVER PERCENTAGE

At Stage Four, it would be another 20% of responsibility handed back to the resident. This would be usually around the 10-month mark of the program.

TOTAL RESIDENT CONTROL — 85%

By this stage, the resident has a lot of independence to make choices in their own lives and are generally working four days per week, Tuesday to Friday. Now that they are at Stage Four, they can move to five days paid work per week. We want to see the resident working hard and building relationships with their families, friends and the community. They will have an 8.30 pm curfew, with more freedom on the weekends.

We consider mentoring to be a vital part of our program. We want to see all senior residents giving back to the program by encouraging the newer residents along and helping to maintain the Shalom culture.

HANDING BACK RESPONSIBILITY

When it come to this Stage of the program, the resident will have a phone and car, so they should begin making their own appointments and looking after all their medical and financial issues. We slowly hand responsibility back to the residents to begin to manage all their entire affairs.

We not only hand it over, but we also teach them what to do. As an organisation, we should have by now sorted out the entirety of their affairs, so now we hand back over that responsibility. That's their myGov account, superannuation, taxation, child support, Medicare, finances medical issues, as well as the responsibility of paying all external debt left that they may have.

So, they should now be in charge of the following aspects of their life:

MYGOV

- Looking after their own finances
- Calendar maintenance — making and keeping their own appointments, including medical ones
- Making sure they book their own mentoring sessions
- Looking after their own receipts for tax purposes and organising their own taxation lodgments and returns
- Paying off their own bills.

ACCOUNTABILITY

It's really important to surround yourself with people you know you can trust to keep you accountable, making sure that they are a good influence in your life, and they will check in on you to see how you're going with all your newfound freedom, so you don't slip up.

Stage Fours should be putting back into those coming behind them. It is also important that they are walking in truth.

As they now have transport and a mobile phone, Stage Fours are responsible for making sure that they look after their own calendar, meaning they have to book their own appointments with their mentor and pay all their own bills.

STAGE FIVE

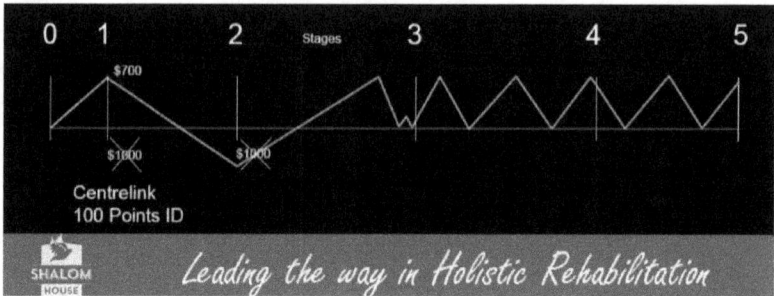

WE HAND OVER PERCENTAGE

At Stage Five, we will have given 14% more control of their life back to the resident. This usually happens to the resident around the 12-month mark of the program.

TOTAL RESIDENT CONTROL — 99%

In Stage Five, the resident can choose to be moved out of a main house and into shared accommodation with other senior residents.

This Stage is a period during which the resident has full control of their life. They are making choices on how to live and what type of life they want to pursue. During this period, we will continue to monitor the resident's progress which may include random drug testing.

The residents are required to demonstrate all of the moral and lifestyle choices that they have learned whilst in the program, to show that they are ready to graduate. How well they cope with the temptations of everyday life and how they interact with their loved ones will determine if they are ready for the next step.

- Working full-time
- They are debt free
- Relationships are restored
- Moving out of Shalom
- Expectations of a Stage 5.

GRADUATION

WE HAND OVER PERCENTAGE
At graduation, it would be the last 1% going back to the resident. This is usually around the 16-month mark of the program.

TOTAL RESIDENT CONTROL — 100% MEANS THE SHALOM HOUSE PROGRAM IS COMPLETED.

Stage	% Transferred in this stage	Total % transferred back to resident
Beginning	5%	5%
One	15%	20%
Two	20%	40%
Three	25%	65%
Four	20%	85%
Five	14%	99%
Graduation	1%	100%

When the resident has demonstrated that they are capable of living free from the program and feels ready to graduate from Shalom, they make an application that asks the resident why they feel ready. We assess each application, speaking with the resident to make sure that a support network is present and that they are set up to fully succeed. We take many things into consideration when approving an application to leave our program. What we want to see is that they are putting into practice everything they were taught at Shalom and being a productive member of the society that they have now entered back into. When a person graduates, we are saying that not only do we support and honour them in what they have achieved, but also that we are confident that they will not go back to their old ways. The resident's graduation is done in the presence of their peers and family and is a major event in the Shalom House family. After graduation, the resident is so well connected in their community and has a wide network of friends, mentors, counsellors and family, so that life simply carries on with a sense of achievement and purpose.

CHAPTER FIFTEEN — SHALOM HOUSE OFFICE DEPARTMENTS

RESIDENT CARE

The Resident Care Department was established to look after every resident's needs from the day they enter the program until they leave. After a successful intake interview, this department will complete the intake process for each resident by working through the Intake Pack. Intake Packs explain to the residents and families about the entirety of the program, not just for the residents but also for their families. These Intake Packs also highlight the expectations we have on both the resident and the families, so that all parties involved know exactly what is expected from them from Day One.

Resident Care Officers are also the first point of contact for all family members throughout a resident's stay. This includes if a family member wants to know any information about how their loved one is going, including any updates on personal or legal matters, until such time where a resident's weekly phone calls commence or if the family member has any concerns regarding the resident's wellbeing. Resident Care also takes care of all after-hours medical emergencies, and collects all new intakes from the airport, prisons and train stations. They also handle the internal mailing system, house communication and job board updates. Every house has an administration area that has various communication slips that can be filled out by the residents to help them communicate with the office, depending on the needs of the residents.

COMMUNICATION SLIPS

These communication slips cover areas such as:

- Doctors
- Dentist
- General Medical
- Home Leave
- Day Leave
- Centrelink Reporting
- Resident Reimbursement
- Goods to be Purchased
- Spends
- Accident Reports
- General department meeting requests.

JOB BOARD

Every house at Shalom has a weekly Jobs Board that shows who and on what days residents are working with and when. This is applicable to Stages Two to Five. It shows the employer's name and day of work, including how many days that they will be working with that employer. This board is updated every week.

Resident Care are also the ones that need to phone family members when a resident exits the program, to inform them that their loved one has left and ensure that everyone is on the same page as to how to help that person, now they have gone.

It is so important to say how they 'need' to be helped, and not in how they 'want' to be helped.

If a resident does leave, Shalom Resident Care tries to assist families to redirect the absent resident back to Shalom to finish what they started and to encourage the family NOT to enable the resident.

We don't want the resident to stay the same as they were, and we also don't want the families to do what they have always done by enabling them. Residents need to be encouraged to finish what they have started, and we don't want families to continue to enable the residents to make wrong choices.

Each House has a Resident Care Officer who completes bag searches, random drug and alcohol urinalysis, car searches, plus monitor the incoming books and DVDs to maintain a positive Shalom culture. They are also responsible for packing a resident's belongings upon exit and communicating with ex-residents to collect their belongings. The Resident Care Department is one of the most important departments of the organisation.

RANDOM TESTS

Random tests are carried out regularly on every resident, including staff.

- Drug test
- Alcohol test
- Nicotine test.

If a positive test does come back, they are either kicked out of the program, restarted (going back to the beginning of the Stages) or they will face some sort of disciplinary action. This all depends on the circumstances of how the positive result was found. For example, did they own up to it without being confronted or was it a surprise random test, where contraband was found, that led to the discovery of a positive test?

RESPONSIBILITIES & DUTIES

- Manage communications, and act as the liaison point, between resident families and Shalom House
- Coordinate communications between the departments in the office and the residents through the mailing system by delivering mail from the office to residents and from residents to the office
- Organise the mail boxes on the properties with the necessary paperwork, distribute paperwork and amend the property whiteboards to reflect residents currently on relevant properties

- File and archive current and former residents' intake information

- Collect and record every new resident's intake information to help direct the relevant office departments on how to handle the resident's needs, e.g., financial matters, Centrelink issues, court appearances and medical needs

- Explain program rules to prospective residents, facilitate signing and ensure any family present at the prospective resident's induction sign the family intake forms

- Arrange each new resident to sign EPOA in favour of Shalom House (to occur as soon as possible after induction) and search new resident's personal property for contraband

- Store confiscated resident property (if not disposed of) and maintain a register of items confiscated, stored or disposed of

- Communicate testimony requests to residents, provide materials to residents to record testimonies and facilitate typing of testimonies (and social media post of testimony if both consented to by the residents and deemed desirable to do so)

- Collect and distribute the property of the residents if they exit the program early and ensure an exit form is filled out in respect of that resident

- Act as liaison point with residents who are no longer in the program

- Draft forms and related paperwork for the residents to communicate with the office

- Attend office meetings to raise and seek resolutions regarding Resident Care Departmental issues

- Liaise between residents and mentors to collate a phone list with approved contacts for residents

- Manage communications between the Shalom House office and the residents including management of Home Leave applications, iPod purchase (including arranging signing of Device Purchase change agreements)

- Manage the digital files for the residents, oversee the administrative data collection for the residents

- Transport residents as required outside of office hours (e.g., an emergency hospital visit provided there are no House leaders available to do the transportation) or picking up interstate residents from WA arrival point (e.g., airport)

- Maintain the Storage Room Registry

- Assist with paperwork and approvals for item drop-offs by residents' families and friends

- Conduct urinalysis for residents in accordance with Shalom House policy or on a randomised basis as instructed by senior management.

ID SERVICES DEPARTMENT

Our ID Services Department helps all residents obtain the essential 100 points of Identification. They prepare all of the external and internal appointments for Shalom House residents, ensuring each resident has the appropriate ID. This means obtaining a birth certificate, driver's licence, Medicare card, bank card, student ID card or even an 18 plus ID card.

Some residents enter Shalom House with very little or no ID. ID Services works in conjunction with other departments and organisations to start the process of gaining 100 points of ID for the resident.

At the two-week mark of the program, the ID Services Department staff member sits down with a resident to work out what ID they do have and where any other ID might be e.g., family and friends. Resident Care would be notified and will contact the relevant people to arrange for the ID to be brought into the office where it will be safely stored.

In most cases, the ID Services Department must make appointments with the Courts, Births, Deaths and Marriages (BDM) or the Department of Transport (DOT) to obtain a new copy of the birth certificate or driver's licence on the person's behalf.

ID Services arrange for an update of a resident's personal details with DOT, Australian Electoral Commission (AEC), banks and Medicare and any other agencies online through the myGov system. This is to ensure that everything is not only up to date, but also that all previous mailing addresses are removed from their systems.

Once the resident has 100 points of ID and has been in the Shalom House program for one month, all residents are then given their ID and wallets back. This provides the resident with a little bit of responsibility, an important part of the program.

RESPONSIBILITIES & DUTIES

- Obtain 100 points of identification for all Shalom Residents e.g., Birth Certificate, Driver's Licence or Photo ID Card, Medicare Card, Health Care/Pensioner Concession Card and bank statements/cards

- Compile appointment folders with the necessary identification and paperwork enclosed for the scheduled appointments e.g., Doctor & Dentist appointments which will require a Medicare Card and/or Health Care/Pensioner Concession Card

- Communicate with the Movements Department to ensure appointment folders are prepared for the following day's appointments

- Complete Driver's Licence and Demerit Point checks

- Arrange for the return of identification at the one-month mark once 100 points of ID is obtained

- Scan and log incoming and outgoing identification into a resident's file and master spreadsheet

- Update address and contact details with DOT, Medicare, AEC and banks

- Complete and apply for Extraordinary Driver's Licences where necessary and needed

- Apply for Working With Children checks where needed.

- Apply for Birth Certificates and Citizenship Certificates within Australia and overseas

- Daily coordination of transportation and movements for male and female residents to and from appointments, paid work and accompany them to various external organisations e.g., Centrelink, Banks, Doctors, DOT

- Scanning and collating of Stores receipts for the Accounts Department to process.

SOCIAL SERVICES DEPARTMENT

The Social Services Department's primary focus is to set up a resident to not only be able to pay for their own rehabilitation, but also to consolidate every residents' social services to be rolled into one, updated and current.

We do this by creating a myGov ID and getting the residents onto Centrelink's JobSeeker, Disability Support Pension (DSP), Age Pension payments as well as many different pension options to assist Australian Defence Force veterans and their family members through the Department of Veterans' Affairs (DVA).

It's important to remember that Centrelink was set up by our government for a person facing a short-term crisis and not for them to live off in the long term.

If the resident does not already receive Centrelink benefits or needs to update their existing account to be able to pay for their rehabilitation, Shalom House's myGov Department looks after it. They also ensure the resident is receiving the correct payments such as JobSeeker, DSP, Age Pension or a range of DVA pensions and any relevant allowances they may be entitled to.

This depends on what benefit they are receiving, so it's so important for all personal details to be accurate for each resident. Not only do they set up or maintain other myGov linked services such as Medicare (for vaccination status proof), ATO (includes superannuation), Child Support, they bring all those services up to date. Taxation is a prime example. All residents' taxation lodgments are made up to date until the day they entered Shalom.

Another example would be a search of all the superannuation accounts that may be held by any resident is undertaken. Following the findings and communication with the resident, all of their accounts are rolled over into one personal account. This is done with all relevant myGov services such as Child Support, Medicare and others that are listed above.

The Australian Government's myGov system not only manages Centrelink deductions, but they also forward all debt-related information from all the linked services to the Finance Department within Shalom. We also collate additional documents requested by Centrelink and upload these via their portal on the resident's behalf. We liaise between Job Providers and Centrelink for the resident's deductions and debts. We don't use external job search providers as we do everything in-house in the form of our labour hire and Shalom Works crews.

RESPONSIBILITIES & DUTIES

- Create a myGov account for residents and link to the necessary government departments

- Arrange for new residents to apply for and receive Centrelink payments as soon as possible

- Manage Shalom House nominee status and payment destination for each resident's Centrelink payments

- Liaise with Centrelink on behalf of residents where necessary

- Coordinate Centrelink job provider requirements

- Manage Centrelink payment deductions for various third-party payees including court fines, Time To Pay (TTP) arrangements and other debt repayment

- Schedule appointments using the central calendar system for residents to attend Centrelink in person

- Oversee the Stage One, Two and Three residents with reporting earnings to Centrelink including levying of fines against residents for failure to report on time

- Organise superannuation rollovers where residents have multiple superannuation funds requiring consolidation – this can include tracing such funds on behalf of residents

- Facilitate superannuation hardship claims, being the early drawdown of a resident's super fund upon grounds of hardship

- Update Social Services and residents' folders and Excel spreadsheets as needed

- File and manage Centrelink, Child Support, ATO and superannuation communication on behalf or residents if required

- Equip and assist Stage Four residents to self-manage Centrelink and other myGov services so that Shalom House office assistance is no longer required

- Represent the Social Services Department at Office Meetings

- Manage staff/volunteers in the Social Services Department

- Provide reports/updates to the Office Manager.

MEDICAL DEPARTMENT

The Medical Department aims to foster the good health and wellbeing of the residents by managing their entire medical, dental and complementary issues, to obtain the best healthcare outcomes within the program for all residents. After a successful intake, the Medical Department completes a full medical assessment to obtain pre-existing conditions and information regarding their life controlling issues that may require medical attention. This includes a full medical examination as well as blood and urine samples. The Medical Department also coordinates appointments with the General Practitioner and Psychiatrist who work closely with our residents to provide them with adequate care.

If a resident has a medical issue that they wish to get seen to, they communicate with the Medical Department via a communication note available on all properties, and appointments are made according to their level of urgency. We treat all medical conditions as advised by the medical professionals and in accordance with the Shalom Program.

FINANCE DEPARTMENT

The Finance Department's goal is to identify outstanding debts of all residents, regardless of the money being a personal debt or a credit agency debt. They have a major responsibility to assist each resident to achieve their debt-free status, something all residents MUST achieve before they can graduate.

This process commences at the initial finance appointment held around the two-week mark of the resident's program. This interview with the resident is to obtain a comprehensive overview of their financial position. Outstanding debts with all financial and credit institutions: car and personal loans, mortgages, overdrafts, government agency debts (Child Support, Centrelink & ATO), service providers (Telstra, Synergy & council rates). Reimbursing family and friends who are owed money by the resident are also part of this process.

At the three-month mark, we apply to put all outstanding fines of the resident onto a Time-To-Pay arrangement or community service. The reason we wait until the three-month mark is that we want to have peace of mind that the resident actually intends to complete our program. There is nothing worse than beginning this time-consuming process by letting all credit providers know where they are and also starting to put in place payment arrangements, and then have the resident leave. The first debt that we endeavour to repay is the intake fee that may have been paid by a member of the family or friend. This is a vital part of a resident's program and the first stage in taking financial ownership of their lives. More often than not, a resident has never repaid any money they borrowed, so taking ownership of their finances starts here.

We also organise a Volunteer Police Clearance Report to obtain their criminal history and a Financial Credit Report from Equifax or Baycorp to obtain any legal debts that they may not be aware of. Once the essential financial information is obtained, we communicate with relevant creditors to freeze outstanding debts and explore hardships options until the resident's six-month mark of the program.

At this time, another appointment is held with the resident to set financial goals such as saving and budgeting funds, working towards being 100 percent debt free. This is generally achieved by the resident starting paid work from Stage Two of the program. We can commence negotiating debt settlement offers once funds start coming in and are available with substantial discounts, sometimes resulting in debt waivers. The Finance Department also deals with real estate agencies to finalise leases and tenancies for residents when they enter the program or arrange for homeowners to have their homes cleaned and leased out.

PROGRAM MANAGER

The Program Manager is responsible for ensuring each department is on target to complete the practical aspects of the program for each resident, e.g., Centrelink, ID, Directions and Finance. The Program Manager utilises the 'board' which is detailed information on each resident written on a whiteboard, and 'popplets,' a mind map application we use on our smart devices to administratively provide a visual overview of the resident's program. The Program Manager's job is to also make sure that various departments act on the resident's behalf, depending on the length of time they have been in the program, as well as the Stage of the program that they are at.

All departments, before initiating anything on any resident's behalf on any matter, must get their action signed off by the Program Manager for accountability, such as ID Services, myGov, Centrelink, Directions, Finances and Medical must have the Program Manager sign off on every item prior to it being actioned.

OFFICE MANAGER

The Office Manager oversees all departments, especially the Program Manager, who oversees each department to ensure they are running efficiently and in accordance with Shalom's standard operating procedures. The Office Manager provides support to staff in all departments and training of staff when required. They also monitor the resident trust accounts to ensure there are sufficient funds to cover the cost of their rent each week as well as medical and general living expenses. They must be the final sign-off person for:

- Notes from residents to various departments
- Home and day leave forms
- Phone number approvals
- Staff leave forms and Staff /Resident reimbursements
- External Invoices to be paid
- Police Clearances requests
- Financial Credit Reports
- Resident spending amounts along with Stage changes
- Update all residents trust information.

The Management Department must oversee all work carried out by the Program Manager and other departments to ensure the correct level of accountability is in place. It is also the Management Department's job to coordinate with the Movements Department to ensure efficient transportation for all residents to appointments including getting to paid work. It is also Management that receives all incoming communication mail and notes by reviewing them before forwarding to the respective departments or person.

FINANCE DEPARTMENT RESPONSIBILITIES & DUTIES

- Meet with new residents to obtain a comprehensive overview of their financial position

- Arrange for an EPOA to be signed by each resident authorising the Finance Department to act in their best interests

- Order and analyse Equifax or Baycorp credit checks

- Order a National Police Clearance Certificate

- Record and file all information (including any relevant documentation) in relation to a resident's outstanding debts with all financial and credit institutions, government agencies and service providers

- Contact the Fines Enforcement Registry (FER) regarding resident outstanding fees or infringements, pending legal proceedings or applicable bail restrictions

- Collaborate with residents' creditors to request freezing outstanding debt and explore hardship options and/or discounted settlements

- Transfer of fines to a Time to Pay order (TTP) through Centrelink's Centrepay system

- Updating the Excel spreadsheet of Resident Finances' Master Sheet as relevant

- Registering certain residents for a Work Development Order through Community Corrections and monitoring/recording community service hours completed by every resident

- Monitoring all debt payment arrangements and ensuring timely payment

- Recommending and providing information to residents on bankruptcy in certain instances (and with relevant approvals)

- Mentoring and encouraging residents to wisely manage their finances, including budgeting training

- Liaising with Community Corrections about post-sentencing requirements/orders, reporting or Work Development Orders

- Assisting with the sale of a resident's assets to meet financial obligations including houses and cars or facilitating rental of property assets

- Liaising with Child Support and other government agencies to reduce outstanding resident debts

- Coordinating with residents' partners to assist with bill payment and general financial management

- Communicating with banks and organisations in different countries

- Dealing with and arranging tax returns and taxation matters to be brought up to date

- Handling, maintaining and obtaining income protection insurance

- Assisting residents with issues relating to any businesses they may hold, including continuation, maintenance or liquidation.

MOVEMENTS DEPARTMENT

RESPONSIBILITIES & DUTIES

- Daily coordination of the transportation and movements of male and female residents to and from appointments, paid work and accompany them to various external organisations: Centrelink, Banks, Doctors & DOT

- Transport and accompany residents during office hours to any emergency hospital visits necessary

- Communicate with other internal departments to ensure appointments don't conflict with other appointments, keeping in mind locations, transport options and personnel availability

- Make Calendar appointments and enter information onto the work schedule for all residents

- Coordinate drivers and volunteer drivers

- Review appointment folders to ensure all necessary identification is enclosed, and the resident's bank card is booked out if needed on the day

- Re-fuelling of Shalom House vehicles

- Collection of pre-starts and forwarding them to the Mechanical Department

- Organise cleaning of vehicles to a high standard

- Drafting weekend schedule to allocate drivers

- Reporting vehicle defects

- Collection of pharmacy medications for the Medical Department

- Transportation of weekly urinalysis samples to the pathology for processing

- Arrange for reimbursement of transportation costs from the residents for paid work

- Organise and prepare vehicle and drivers for tours.

MEDICAL DEPARTMENT

RESPONSIBILITIES & DUTIES

- Meet with new residents to undertake a New Resident Medical Intake as a means of gauging their physical and mental health status at time of intake

- Organise initial medical appointment with Shalom House-approved general practitioner for routine bloods and urine testing, obtaining pathology forms and for a Medical Certificate for Centrelink

- Addressing the individual medical issues of each resident according to their specific needs and requirements as informed by their medical intake and by subsequent resident communications

- To book all necessary appointments with allied health professionals, hospitals and general practitioner

- Liaising with Movements, Directions, ID Services and the resident in question within Shalom House and with the external agencies

- Ensure all necessary referrals and completed questionnaires are provided for each appointment

- Update the resident's Excel Medical Master Sheet and their Medication Management Spreadsheet

- Pharmacy runs to obtain medications (prescription and over-the-counter) as per Shalom House directives

- Make up Webster Packs for those residents requiring regular medications over a prolonged period of time

- Deliver all medications to the residents at their respective houses

- Sufficient medications available in the safe for those residents requiring the same, and that there are prescriptions on hand to replenish such medications when the time comes

- Work in liaison with Health & Safety following on-site, work-related and Workers' Compensation injuries

- Handle all incoming mail relating to medical matters for residents, including follow-up appointments and outstanding accounts for medical services provided.

- Providing medical advice and information as required

- Report Medical 'red' incidents to upper management.

- Function as point of contact for all Medical matters for all residents in Shalom House, as a representative of the residents and as an ambassador for Shalom House to all external medical agencies

- Maintain hard-copy records (filing) and complete other general administrative duties as required

- Attend and participate as required in weekly office meeting

- Observe all safe working practices and work as directed by your supervisor

- Ensure that you take reasonable care to ensure your own safety and health at work and that of others

- Undertake duties and responsibilities in accordance with Shalom House policies and procedures and demonstrate expected behaviours aligned with the Shalom Employee Handbook / Volunteer Handbook

- Demonstrate a basic understanding of Shalom House's risk management processes.

- Perform other duties as directed by upper management such as Chief of Staff or CEO

- Manage emotions and actions appropriately and professionally

- Be an effective team member

- Build appropriate and professional relationships with others, using appropriate communication skills to ensure that people understand your message

- Look to continually develop self and others to improve performance

- Look at the bigger picture presently and in the future, understanding Shalom House and the surrounding environment

- Use appropriate decision-making processes that consider outcomes and implications

- Set objectives and manage self, time and resources in working towards them.

SAFETY DEPARTMENT

RESPONSIBILITIES & DUTIES

- Maintain the Training Matrix to keep a record of all qualifications of residents to ensure each resident is qualified/trained for any work they may complete

- Appoint First Aid Officers, train and display names/contact details where applicable

- Shalom Labour Works Client Visits to make sure the client workplace is a safe environment for all residents:
    — Ensure the completion of a Client Visit Log Form and any necessary follow-up
    — Record the Client Visit in the Client Visit Log Excel spreadsheet

- Ensure other departments and workers are completing work in a safe manner

- Bring correction and implement controls where work is being completed in a manner that is not safe

- Respond to incidents and accidents, ensuring appropriate incident reports are completed, review the incident where required and implement controls

- Participate in weekly Shalom Works meetings, presenting all incidents for the week, a toolbox talk/safety topic and any issues from the week that need to be raised

- Maintenance of safety records, including scanning and filing including:
  - Training Matrix
  - WHS Register & Risk Register
  - Safety Communication Log
  - Incident Report Live Note
  - Safety Equipment Register
  - Client Visit Log

- Present safety issues from the week at the Leadership Meetings including any concerns about residents, changes to procedures and issues that will be raised at the Recalibration Meeting for that week

- Present toolbox talks to the entire organisation on a monthly basis at Recalibration Meetings, ensuring a Toolbox Talk Attendance Record form is completed by all staff, volunteers and residents

- Present safety issues to the entire organisation at Recalibration Meeting on a weekly basis

- Convert Recalibration Live Note into Recalibration Minutes according to an established format for records

- Keep records of the Stores (Block) Sign-in/Sign-out forms by scanning and filing as well as providing new forms as needed

- Create and provide Tag-Out tags to Stores (Block) and Shalom Works trucks for damaged equipment

- Oversee training for residents and staff:
    - — White Cards at the 8-week mark
    - — Manual Handling Training at the 8-week mark
    - — First Aid Training for residents and staff/volunteer leadership
    - — Other training as requested by residents and approved by the COO

- Oversee High Risk Work Licence renewals and transfers

- Record all Stores (Property Maintenance) SOP Induction forms (Planer, Circular Saw, Docking Saw etc.) as they are completed in the Store SOP Induction Log spreadsheet

- Source lost tickets/qualifications for residents at the request of the resident, via Directions

- Organise internal Chainsaw or Quick Cut training including obtaining approvals, scheduling, providing course materials and providing cards once course is successfully completed.

- Prepare agreements, questionnaires, training cards, waivers, policies and similar documentation, maintaining and updating these documents as required.

- Write Safety Procedures as required, ensuring new procedures are circulated and implemented properly

- Ensure Resident Induction processes are followed:
    — Block Induction as soon as possible following a resident entering the program
    — Shalom Works Induction, sent home at the 4-week mark
    — Shalom Labour Works Induction, computer-based when a resident achieves Stage Two
    — Shalom Works Truck Leader Induction, when a resident is elected as Shalom Works Truck Leader
- Work alongside the Medical Department when needed to properly manage incidents
- Maintain First Aid kits in houses, trucks and all work areas, including completing a 6-monthly stock take of the first aid items in the cupboard in the breezeway
- Oversee Take Fives as completed by Shalom Works Trucks and Property Maintenance Trucks. Review, scan and file once completed
- Oversee resident cleaners who attend the office on Tuesdays and Thursdays, ensuring they remain on task and cleaning is completed to a high standard
- Make sure all PPE is being worn where applicable
- Create and maintain emergency evacuation procedures and posters, coordinating evacuation/emergency responses and organise evacuation drills once per year
- Ensure fire extinguishers and fire blankets are serviced on a yearly basis

- Create and implement Safe Work Method Statements (SWMS) for high risk work

- Engage in regular consultation with management, other employees and residents regarding stringent safety and risk management

- Implementing risk management procedures and incident reporting procedures and training residents and staff in these procedures

- Assess Incident Reports for quality and ensure they are completed to a high standard

- Completing site inspections of Shalom.

On all Properties:

- Install safety signs where required

- Maintain Safety Data Sheet file at the Office (cleaning products etc.) and the Block while ensuring the SDS for new hazardous chemicals are added to the SDS file.

PROGRAM MANAGER

RESPONSIBILITIES & DUTIES

- The purpose and objective of the Program Manager's role is to oversee and facilitate the progress of every resident through all Stages from intake to graduation
- Ensure issues regarding a resident's recovery are processed and dealt with at appropriate times:
  — Intake payment is paid back first
  — At the 2-month mark, a White Card & their Direction is completed
  — At the 3-month mark, fines are put on a Time to Pay arrangement or court fines are converted to a Work Development Order.
- Mission statement of the Program Manager: "Don't let anyone slip through the gaps."
- The popplet program is used to store relevant information for the resident's progress, mapping their Stages, outstanding issues and highlighting any requirements for progress
- The Resident Board is a vital tool to oversee a resident's movements in the program and needs to be updated regularly to avoid miscommunication
- Regularly (Weekly at least) meet with the Office Manager (OM) to go over the Resident Board to identify high-priority residents and tasks to be delegated and followed up with departments.

- The Program Manager should be looking for key issues in a resident's life that need to be actioned to progress them quickly through the program.
- Facilitate banking transactions including receipt of funds from Men's Shed, church tithes, intake fees and all other cash which are to be logged into money book and banked with Shalom House's financial institution
- Retrieve mail from Shalom House PO Box and distribute to relevant departments
- Retrieve mail from CEO PO Box and deliver to the CEO or Chief of Staff.

OFFICE MANAGER

RESPONSIBILITIES & DUTIES
- Oversee residents' trust accounts to ensure they are receiving Centrelink Payments, trust account top-ups for rent, program expenses are paid, invoices from Medical and Finance Department payments processed
- Liaise with residents regarding payment of their rent and any monies owed to Shalom House.
- Ensure all office departments are running efficiently and smoothly by ensuring office operations and procedures are organised, correspondence is monitored, filing systems are designed and followed
- Monitor procedures for record keeping
- Monitor clerical, administrative and secretarial responsibilities and tasks amongst staff

- Offer support and guidance to the Heads of departments within the office, mentor and train them in their leadership roles
- Coordinate office activities for maximum efficiency
- Function as the up-line for all office departments, including resolving queries and conflict resolution between staff/volunteers
- Present corporate issues about office administration to residents at weekly Recalibration meetings
- Liaise with Chief of Staff regarding performance management of staff and volunteers within the office
- Monitor departmental goals and objectives and ensure targets are being met
- Administration of bills and notes to be reviewed and signed off by Executive Officer including resident notes or office forms within the following categories: resident money requests, superannuation payout requests, tax return applications, closure of resident trust accounts, fuel reimbursements, bills, Home Leave requests, resident exit forms and staff leave request forms
- Receipt of resident Equifax credit files from Finance & Legal Affairs Department.
- Facilitate individual credit file reviews by CEO to obtain authorisation for further action as required by the Finance & Legal Affairs Department
- Train and work alongside the Program Manager to update the resident information boards and resident files (hard and soft copy media to keep track of resident progress and provide a high-level overview)

- Undertake duties and responsibilities in accordance with Shalom policies and procedures and demonstrate expected behaviours aligned with the Shalom Employee Handbook/Volunteer Handbook
- Demonstrate an adequate understanding of Shalom House's risk management processes
- Coordinate and take the lead of office staff meetings on Monday mornings
- Ensure results are measured against standards while coming up with solutions and necessary changes to be presented to Chief of Staff along the way
- Ensure security, integrity and confidentiality of data
- Oversee adherence to office policies and procedures
- Perform other duties as directed
- Manage emotions and actions appropriately and professionally
- Build appropriate and professional relationships with others using appropriate communication skills to ensure that people understand your message
- Look to continually develop self and others to improve performance
- Look at the bigger picture presently and in the future
- Understand Shalom House and the surrounding environment
- Use appropriate decision-making processes that consider outcomes and implications
- Set objectives and manage self, times and resources in working towards them.

HOUSE RULES

- Respect Everyone
- Obey Leadership
- No Swearing
- No Lies
- No Gossiping
- No Stealing
- No Fighting
- Have Integrity
- Be Honest
- Make Good Choices
- Have a Good Attitude.

First in Charge Role — 1ic
- Follow the instructions of the Red leader
- Disciple 2ic and housemates
- Liaise with 2ic regularly to maintain House order and culture, run house meetings with all 1ic's being at House meetings on Wednesdays/Saturdays
- House inductions
- Mentor referrals to Red Leader
- Discipling and correction
- Training and equipping
- Housemate personal hygiene
- Maintaining Shalom culture, leading by example
- Duty of care
- Overseeing morning devotionals

- Uphold Stage rules with housemates (ensure Stage Threes and Fours are putting back into the house)
- Know which housemates are on or off the property at any time
- Advise 2ic when you are on or off the property
- Dealing with heart issues
- Communicating behavioural and House issues to the Red Leader.

Second in Charge Role — 2ic
- Disciple 3ic and delegate jobs to them where necessary
- Bus head checks
- Pair up new fellas for all church services and events
- Ensuring all housemates are ready 10 minutes early and outside
- for all church services and events
- Organise and oversee house cleans
- Inspecting jobs upon completion
- Ensuring all beds and rooms are neat and tidy
- Centrelink report reminders
- Ensure House is locked up and lights/fans/air cons are turned off
- Oversee communication with the Storeman for food and chemical needs
- Answer ALL House-related questions
- Communicate with the 1ic in regard to the behaviour/attitude and work ethic of all housemates
- Work with the 1ic to ensure Shalom House culture is being followed

- Lead by example
- Ensure all housemates are clean shaven before all church services and events
- Advise 1ic when residents are on or off the property
- Ensure all cooking is undertaken while using gloves
- Delegate jobs and organise cooking rosters
- Prepare worklists
- Make sure lights are off at the end of every night.

All Residents' Role
- Setting up their rooms
- Help new residents to feel welcome
- Introduce them to their roommates
- Talk them through the process of keeping their rooms clean and tidy
- Explain that we respect each other's space and privacy
- Show the resident which drawers, shelves and hanging space they can use.

Introductions
- Take them through the House, introducing them one by one to the other residents in the House
- Tell the new resident that they don't need to remember all the names straight away as it may take some time.

Leadership Model
- Teach them how the Shalom authority model works, what the roles are of the House Leaders, 1ic's and 2ic's
- Introduce the resident to the Leaders in the House and their roles (1ic and 2ic, explaining 1ic is for heart issues and 2ic is House issues).

Food
- Show the resident where they can store their food and which of the fridges are communal or private
- Explain hygienic food preparation practices and the need to wear gloves during cooking to maintain strict OH&S standards
- Show the resident where the plates, pots, cups, mugs and pantry are in the House.

Laundry
- Describe how to use the washing machine, explaining how we don't use hot water to wash our clothes
- Show them where the washing powder is stored and where to hang their washing
- Explain that we don't leave washing on the line longer than necessary because others need to use the lines.

Chores
- Explain the chores board/cooking roster, highlighting how it is residents' responsibility to maintain a clean and tidy living environment, not leaving things scattered around when we leave a room.

Mail Box

- Explain that the mail box is to be checked every day so the office can help the resident efficiently
- Explain how to use the communication slips e.g., daily communications, essential Centrelink reporting, family belonging drop offs and Home Leaves
- Explain how medical requests work, highlighting the need to be specific with the illness to assist with the department's decision-making process.

Devotionals

- Show the resident how to find books in the Bible using a Table Of Contents and how to use the Daily Bread
- Explain the minimum of thirty-minute devotional times first thing in the morning before showering and having breakfast
- Offering a brief explanation on why it is important to read devotionals.

Lights on and off

- Explain the times the resident can stay up, not making too much noise
- If the resident can't sleep, point them to the 1ic
- Explain who would be waking them up in the morning, what time they would be woken up.

House Clean
- Explain the daily house cleaning chores as well as the Wednesday and Saturday major House cleans
- Explain to the new resident what their job is and talk them through how to do it, get their job checked off by the 2ic who oversees the house cleans.

Money
- How to order money on a Wednesday
- How much the resident can have at any one time
- Explain that we don't lend or borrow money to or from other residents or anyone else
- No selling possessions.

Working Week
- Explain what the working week looks like, Monday to Friday including Recalibration
- Explain why we wear work gear (safety boots, hi-vis)
- Help the resident to get any items of clothing that they might be missing, must have steel-cap boots

Where residents can go, what they can do
- Explain why we stay in our own Houses and don't wander into other Houses
- Where the boundaries of the property are
- Explain why they aren't allowed into other people's rooms.

Sunday Shopping

- Explain to the resident what they can and can't buy
- Tell the resident clearly that they can't buy medications, energy drinks, supplements or magazines.

Communications, non-negotiables

- Explain what to avoid talking about
- How we deal with conflict
- Emphasise that we don't gossip or slander
- Highlight the importance of being transparent, open and honest about issues.

Buddy System

- In the first month, new residents are to be partnered when attending events, shopping and church
- Explain why we partner them up for the first month.

Centrelink Reporting

- Show the resident where the reporting roster is and point out an example of how they report
- Explain to the resident that they are obliged to report even if they aren't working yet
- Make it clear that they get 4 strikes (1st fail—amnesty, 2nd fail—$45, 3rd fail—$90 and 4th fail—$150 as well as a restart of the program).

ACCOUNTS DEPARTMENT

The Accounts Department manages all income and expenditures for Resident Trust Accounts and all WASG accounts. This includes managing Payroll and Audit requirements.

Accounts is responsible for all areas relating to financial reporting and for developing and maintaining accounting principles, practices and procedures to ensure that accurate and timely financial statements are done. The Accounting Manager also supervises staff and is responsible for managing the team to ensure that work is properly allocated and completed in a timely and accurate manner. The Accounts Department addresses tight deadlines and a multitude of accounting activities including general ledger preparation, financial reporting, year-end audit preparation and the support of budget and forecast activities. Accounts will have contact with senior-level staff and the organisation's Chief Executive Officer and Accountant to guarantee a high level of accountability.

RESPONSIBILITIES & DUTIES

The Accounts Department is always on the go, such as:

- Obtain and maintain a thorough understanding of the financial reporting and general ledger structure
- Ensure an accurate and timely monthly, quarterly and year-end close
- Ensure the timely reporting of all monthly financial information
- Oversee the daily banking requirements

- Ensure the accurate and timely processing of payroll and pay transactions
- Check monthly/quarterly Bank Compliance activities are performed in a timely and accurate manner
- Support budget and forecasting activities
- Collaborate with the other departmental managers to support overall department goals and objectives
- Monitor and analyse department work to develop more efficient procedures and use of resources while maintaining a stringent level of accuracy
- Advise staff regarding the handling of non-routine reporting transactions
- Respond to inquiries from the Chief Executive Officer, Accountant and other managers regarding financial results, special reporting requests and the like
- Work with the Accountant to ensure a clean and timely year-end audit
- Supervise the general ledger group to ensure all financial reporting deadlines are met
- Develop and implement new procedures and features to enhance the workflow of the department
- Provide training to new and existing staff as needed
- Handle personnel issues relating to finance staff conflicts, absenteeism, performance issues, etc.
- Work with direct reports to establish goals and objectives every year and monitor and advise on progress to enhance staff professional development.
- Support CEO and Accountant with special projects and workflow process improvements.

FAMILIES

Families work closely with a resident's spouse/ex-partners/family or DCP with the view to reunite a resident with their child/children, along with various levels of custody arrangements.

MENTORING / COUNSELLING DEPARTMENT

Mentors work closely with a resident to identify and work through life-controlling issues that led them to Shalom House in the first place. Mentors facilitate reconciliation between family members, ex-partners and other loved ones.

We have a qualified Psychiatrist, Psychologist, Counsellors and many mentors on board. All new residents will see a doctor within 72 hours maximum of entering Shalom, even sooner if the doctor is not booked out. We have a psychiatrist who comes in every Wednesday who talks with the residents who require his services. All residents who have been identified as needing to see a psychiatrist will do so ASAP at the psychiatrist's office, after first getting a referral from Shalom House's GP.

We always work with the doctor or any other medical professionals when it comes to the safe administration of medications. Our doctors and psychiatrist are extremely cautious when handing out S8 medications and we will follow their instructions.

The Mentoring/Counselling Department is also responsible for the mental health, emotional care and wellbeing of all residents and staff by way of mentoring/counselling at Shalom House. This is hosted as a therapeutic and holistic model, working collaboratively with all internal departments, external support agencies and supporting medical professionals such as General Practitioners, Doctors, Psychologists, Psychiatrists, etc.

Additionally, Shalom House works with external stakeholders such as the Midvale Hub who provide government-funded and required courses for parents such as the 'Circle of Security,' and 'Tuning into Kids,' etc.

The Head of this department is required to liaise between the Mentors and CEO as required. The CEO or Head of Mentors only allocate residents to mentors. This is in order to match residents with mentor skill sets and experience e.g., addictions, trauma, self-harm etc. All Mentors' caseloads and rosters are always to be considered prior to any new resident allocations.

Mentors are required to work collaboratively with all parties, including office staff for appointments, works staff for both internal and external employment, risk assessments e.g., factoring suitability to operate machinery, operate as a team, operate free from the influence etc. Mentors regularly meet with the residents to facilitate counselling and to further develop relationships with the residents to establish trust.

All Mentors are to be qualified or working towards relevant qualifications with appropriate counselling and ministry experience. Mentors cannot mentor out of their own brokenness, life experience does play a large part in mentoring. This common-sense approach is well received by residents, far more than someone who comes to work with the residents who just has book or head knowledge.

As a Mentor at Shalom House, you come alongside residents with discipling, counselling, teaching, prayer ministry and are involved with the restoration of relationships and families by way of reconciliations. The Mentors are responsible for the reconciliation process, working alongside all parties to facilitate the restoration of broken family units.

The Mentoring/Counselling Department refers couples or prospective couples to couples' counselling hosted weekly by the Marriage Counselling Team who work collaboratively with the allocated Mentors.

MENTOR PA DUTIES
The Mentoring/Counselling Department's PA is to receive condensed notes from the Mentors after each session and ensure Mentors complete and provide notes in a timely manner. The PA updates the Master shared note, adding Stage/New Intake Name/Date of Intake/Date of last contact by the Mentor.
*Note — New intakes must be seen by a Mentor prior to the first weekend of intake.

Up-line Red

If a resident displays any type of mental health behaviour requiring attention, unusual behaviours, expresses any self-harm behaviours, any other serious behavioural issues, or any bad news which could be passed on to another resident that would upset their mood, etc.

All Up-line Red Mentor notes are to be brought to the Head of Mentors as well as the Duty Mentor if on a weekend. Escalate to the CEO if something doesn't feel right or there's elevated concerns from the Mentor, House or Workplace.

External Mail

Read and review any correspondence upon receipt or dispatch ensuring content is appropriate and will not trigger any receiving party. Photograph all notes, pictures, cards, books, correspondence, etc. Send to the relevant Mentor for approval before dissemination to residents.

Resident Enquiry Forms

Write the text date, sign initials, and Mentor initials in the top left-hand corner. Photograph any resident enquiries that come in and text or email them to the Mentor. After they have been sent to the Mentor, place the enquiry form in the relevant mentor's inbox/tray. Keep all correspondence until any concerns have been resolved. Follow up as required. Photos are to be retained to provide evidence that enquiries have been actioned.

Photograph all letters, cards books etc. and text to the Mentor for approval. Process/approve as requested by Mentor (in a Mentors' absence). Books, photos and letters that have been approved are to be sent to the resident.

Check through Home Leave forms for correct dates, times and situations. Highlight anything out of the usual that the Mentors need to be aware of. Liaise with Resident Care and Mentors as required. Approve on behalf of the Mentor if they request it.

Home Leave forms must be submitted at least 14 days prior to the leave going ahead unless exceptional circumstances have been approved. Day Leave is assessed on a case-by-case basis. Home Leave forms are to be placed in the Resident Care tray if approved by the Mentor, then Families Coordinator.

All other approved notes are to be placed in the tray on the Office Manager's desk for the CEO or Families Coordinator for approval.

Oversee the Counselling offices to ensure they are not overcrowded or overbooked and for accountability. Staff are not to mentor a resident of the opposite sex unless another staff member is present in the immediate vicinity.

Check over and initial Reconciliations and popplets before the Mentors take them to the Families Coordinator or the CEO.

Take them to the Families Coordinator or the CEO on behalf of the Mentors if requested. File reconciliation paperwork if completed and successful.

Check the work schedule to reduce double bookings. Manage/oversight on Mentors' appointments and bookings. Liaise with department heads to ensure cohesive scheduling. Work closely with Shalom Works, Directions, Medical and the Mentors to achieve harmony.

Maintain agenda and notes in preparation for fortnightly Mentors' meetings. Record issues to discuss at the fortnightly Mentors meeting.

Record concerns from the Mentors from these meetings. Discuss with the Families Coordinator and CEO as required. Email feedback and meeting minutes to the Mentors.

It is important to read these notes before sending to ensure they make sense and to ensure they are up to date on resident progress and behaviours. Follow up with the House Leaders for clarification before the notes are emailed.

The House Leaders will send separate notes for sensitive issues, these are to be sent to the individual Mentors as required. House Leaders will identify residents who present as 'Up-line-Red' and need mentoring including a brief summary as to why. A Duty Mentor will be allocated as a priority, pending availability.

These notes are to be texted directly to the individual Mentor also. Reds are to be up-lined to the Families Coordinator or Red of Reds immediately. Ensure that the Wage Timesheet is filled out and all accurate hours are provided to Accounts by the end of pay week.

PSYCHIATRIST

Psychiatrist receives referrals for those diagnosed with mental health issues and those who wish to withdraw from prescription medications and helps us manage this process. Psychiatrist is to up-line to the Families Coordinator any residents the mentor feels may benefit from seeing the Psychiatrist, either at his clinic in a formal psychiatrist appointment or at the office or café e.g. if they are hearing voices, acting out of character or showing suicidal ideation. Please Cc the CEO and Families Coordinator in on any of these. Bookings for the Psychiatrist are to be completed via Calendar Invite weekly, alternating one week on and week off for female residents then for male residents.

Bookings are for 30 minutes only. Send all House notes for residents seeing Dr Willem at least 24 hours prior to appointments. Liaise via email with the Psychiatrist about any significant issues regarding residents and also about any late changes to residents' appointments. Significant psychological issues regarding residents should be booked in directly at the Psychiatrist Office for full sessions and not via Shalom appointments onsite.

DOCTORS

GP's provide general medical management to all residents for pre-existing medical conditions, review and manage new illnesses and conditions, issue medical certificates and referrals to other medical services.

PSYCHOLOGIST

The Psychologist works to observe and interpret how our residents relate to one another, then advises our Mentoring Team.

SHALOM WORKS

Some time back, I started a business called 'Shalom Works' which does all types of building maintenance and construction. One hundred percent of the income earned by Shalom Works goes into the running of the Shalom House program. We are not costing the government a cent and what we are doing is working at changing lives.

Shalom House is 'Leading the way in Holistic Rehabilitation.'

The Shalom Works business undertakes work within the community not just to produce a supplementary income to help support the Shalom House program, but also to provide a safe place where all residents can learn new skills and to help them find employment direction for their lives. This business runs primarily to make money for Shalom, but also to provide the residents with the opportunity to learn new skills and assist them with their reintegration into the community.

Our focus is on changing lives, not on making money. It has been hard for us running so many businesses while keeping focused on the rehabilitation of the residents. When you mix rehabilitation and business, it's like mixing politics and religion, it becomes one-sided.

We offer the following services: Softscapes, Hardscapes, Removals as well as Paving & Limestone, Bags of Rags, Secondhand Furniture, Shalom Digital, Furniture Removals, community services etc. These businesses are not only for residents to go out and try their hand at new skills, but also help the residents get used to doing normal work, getting out of bed, making lunches, giving the employers their best during work hours and setting a normal routine.

Property Maintenance

Our Property Maintenance Teams are responsible for the upkeep of the gardens at all of Shalom House's residential properties. They mow, trim and edge the lawns, performing weeding, spreading mulch and pruning all the shrubbery as well as cleaning the gutters and looking after paved areas.

Softscapes

Our Softscapes Teams carry out all types of gardening and landscaping service tasks such as reticulation repair, tree lopping, tree pruning, lawn mowing and slashing, hedge-trimming and shrub-shaping, weeding and mulching, yard clean-ups, garden makeovers, green waste removal and more.

Hardscapes

Our Hardscapes Team installs decking, screens, build awnings, construct pergolas, patios, lean-to areas and other external jobs to do with building maintenance and construction.

Removals

The Removals Teams carry out all types of furniture removal or office moves, and anything in between. We have a number of vehicles set up to move any item across the metro area.

Fencing

Our Fencing Team carries out the removal and installation of all types of fencing from Colorbond, HardieFence, rural and general fencing.

Paving & Limestone

Our Paving & Limestone Team provides all the following services: construction, relaying and repairs to all paving, limestone & retaining walls, paving repairs, relays, or a limestone wall built, brick paving, limestone walls, footpaths, concrete paving, stone paving, driveway, cross overs, repairs or brand-new installations.

Shalom Digital

Shalom Digital is passionate about delivering client-focused services. Their first objective is to establish a genuine relationship with the client, getting to know them and their business goals. Open lines of communication coupled with honesty and integrity are paramount to achieving any level of success. They have a team of people who are experts in their fields. The Website Design and Development Team builds the client's WordPress website from the ground up whilst the Graphic Designer creates custom elements to suit the business's needs. We also offer Search Engine Optimisation and a Google AdWords service.

Café

The Shalom Ladies Café & Boutique offers an opportunity for all new female residents to learn many new skills: catering, cooking, baking, food preparation, commercial food calculations, barista duties, customer service, cash register sales and more. It is an exceptional chance for the ladies who have never worked before to learn to deal with the public face-to-face and to do so on a highly professional, commercial basis.

Secondhand Furniture

Shalom House sells a wide range of secondhand donated furniture and household items: beds, cupboards, tables and chairs, lounge suites and more.

All of our goods have been donated to us by the community where we onsell them to the public and then use the funds to pay for the overheads of running the donations section of Shalom. For us, it's not about making money but providing work for our residents as well as the chance for residents to learn new skills.

Believe it or not, moving furniture around without causing any damage can take a great deal of skill, not to mention the customer service side of things when dealing with the public.

Bags of Rags

We have a wide range of rags for sale made up from all different fabrics from white polish cloth to general clean cloth for spillages etc. All the types of rag bags are made up from secondhand clothing domains to Shalom. What we can resell as secondhand clothing, we will, otherwise it gets turned into rags.

Mechanics

Shalom Mechanical is set up mainly to look after Shalom's fleet of vehicles. We have over 68 vehicles: cars, trucks, buses, tractors, trailers and more. It's a great opportunity for residents to try their hand at mechanics, to not only learn the basics of mechanical repairs, but also gives the residents the opportunity to see if this is a career/life direction that they wish to pursue.

Labour Hire

We set up Shalom Labour Hire so that we could provide employment for our residents, making sure that we would abide by Fair Work Australia's labour rate and also to make it easier for a new employer to give various residents an opening to try various types of employment without the employer having to commit to taking on the resident without all the paperwork involved.

By law, if the rate for an unskilled labourer was $22.50 per hour, we would add 30% to that rate. The 30% is broken down to 9.6% super, public liability, workers comp and a 10% handling fee which goes towards covering the wages of the staff member who runs Shalom Labour Hire. The total of $22.50 plus 30% = $29.25. It's impossible for us to make money from that rate, but for us, it's not about making money but covering staff costs and obeying the laws of our land with regards to fair work wages.

TESTIMONIES

I write this book for no other reason other than I care about people, I am not trying to justify any wrongdoing or any person's actions. I sincerely hope this book can help people not only change their lives but also restore their families. I also write this book in the hope that it will equip rehabilitation centres, drug and alcohol service providers and other agencies that are trying to help people caught up in life-controlling issues. Please know that I am not saying that I know it all and that I have got it all right, but I am saying that there may be some useful information that will help you to help others.

Haters will always hate and will approach most things they look at with the aim of highlighting what they don't agree with while disregarding what does work. Please, when reading this book, if you feel there are things I can learn help me to learn, help me to see what I can't see or what I can do better. Let's work together to help others.

Our society has changed considerably over the last 30 years, what was not acceptable back then is now acceptable today, from the content we watch on TV, how we teach our children, freedom of speech, etc. The younger generation may think it's okay, but the older generation can see the damage it is causing to our society. If you look back over history, you will see that it's history repeating itself.

LIAM'S STORY

My name is Liam, born Liam Conneally in Kingston Upon Thames, Surrey, England. I am 38 years old and I am the eldest of four children (two brothers and one sister) to married parents, still together as I write this. My Mum and Dad always did the best they knew how for us kids, helped us when needed and loved us unconditionally. They have always had a bed for us to sleep in if required and food for us to eat when we were hungry.

Dad always worked long hours, so I never felt like I knew him that well, especially as I believe he did not show or share his emotions and feelings. Dad had studied martial arts and was physically very strong. Mum did most of the disciplining of us children, but I developed a strong fear of my dad and a fear of doing anything that would displease him. I was extremely self-critical and insecure. Mum, on the other hand, was always there but was constantly under the pump caring for four children under five years of age. As the eldest, I found myself helping Mum a lot with her responsibilities and found my identity in this role. Through that position of responsibility, I developed self-entitlement issues. Despite having three siblings close in age, I was extremely lonely and constantly seeking affirmation of my self-worth. I felt like I had to perform well or achieve success to receive the attention and acceptance that I was craving on the inside. I often believed that my other siblings were looked upon more favourably.

From the start of primary school, I had an interest in the opposite sex and developed strong, lustful feelings towards girls. I judged them by their appearance, primarily. I developed these thought patterns and behaviours towards my teachers and other grown women too. In Year One, I was rejected by a girl which planted seeds of fear and rejection. Over the years, I saw this grow into a pursuit of acceptance in unhealthy relationships. My behaviour ranged from flirtatious to controlling, manipulative actions fuelled by those desires and including other shameful habits when no one else was around.

Through this lifestyle, I developed feelings of shame and guilt which I believe I needed to keep to myself, with addiction leading to extreme anxiety which I felt I could just never show anyone. Over time, this developed into even deeper levels of deceitfulness and dishonesty.

Whilst I was generally a good kid at school academically and liked by teachers and fellow students, there were a couple of bullying incidents which I reported but felt like nothing was done about, thus my feelings had not been heard/considered and led to more questioning of my worth and identity. I have never had anyone (partner/best friend) that I have been able to be 100% honest with. I have always felt like I am not worth knowing. The closest I came to a best friend as a child was in the last year of primary school, but at the end of that year, we moved from England to Perth, Australia.

The move itself was exciting but I then felt like I was the odd kid out, completing the last term of Year 7 and then moving up into a high school where all the students already had their cliques. I got to high school and allowed my abilities in sport and music to define my identity, I was neither one of the cool kids or in the nerd kids' groups and found myself in the middle zone, not knowing where I fitted in.

I lusted after the attractive females but was rejected and my craving for sexual intimacy developed as a desire for affirmation. My grades started slipping in Year 10 and I barely graduated Year 12 in 2000. Having been through a Roman Catholic school and struggling, I asked myself, "What's the point of it all?"

I knew of a God and of the Bible but did not know God or feel the Holy Spirit, so I chose to reject religion and would try to do as many extracurricular activities as I could to avoid study and religious activities. I was bullied in Year 8 and never felt like I could stand up for myself, wanting to avoid conflict at all costs but feeling like justice needed to be served, though I just didn't know how, so bottled all these feelings of anger and hurt, bitterness and resentment.

I formed a friendship with two females in Year 10 and we competed in a science project together, being picked to represent our school and coming second in the state. In the following weeks, both females received death threat letters in their mail, addressed to them, signed by someone pretending to be me. I didn't do it, but was framed and unable to clear my name. It ruined my friendships and trust in people and authority figures.

When I eventually had my first girlfriend in Year 11, I was too afraid to make any sexual advancements as I really had no idea what I was doing and feared getting it wrong. She was sexually experienced and attractive. She cheated on me, then dumped me. I hardened my heart, and my fear of rejection grew.

School finished and I started university. I experienced a new kind of freedom. I continued living at home, but I became less accountable, the master of my own universe.

I had made the decision early in my life that I was never going to take recreational drugs. At fourteen, I tasted champagne and made the decision not to drink alcohol, which I have sustained to this day. I know now that this is part of a fear of not being in control. I had to be in control of my life at every single moment. Therefore, I was afraid to be under the influence of a substance.

Through university, I used my controlling, deceptive and manipulative behaviours to navigate several relationships, often more than one at a time. I was looking for love and a heartfelt connection but never found it, so I was never happy or truly filled with joy. I was unfaithful to those whom, I had termed 'my girlfriend'. Still flirtatious and with a confident cover on the outside, I was predatory on the inside, which gave me a sense of invulnerability. I targeted those who were vulnerable and could be controlled. I went through two abortions with one partner and a miscarriage with another.

The burden of my shame and guilt was increasing but I kept that all to myself.

I met the mother of my children at the Midland Gate Shopping Centre and was immediately drawn to the fact that she was a good Christian girl. I was unhappy and aware that I needed to break the cycle of my unfaithfulness and sinful behaviours. The innocence of this good Christian girl was appealing in a way. I felt that I would be able to change, but also that I could control her but not be hurt by her.

We began dating in 2006 and I started going to church with her, serving on the kid's ministry team, partaking in a marriage preparation course, and lying to everyone that I was in it for Jesus. I did not know Him and was not trying to know Him.

We married in 2008 and through our ten and a half years of marriage, I had three high responsibility roles in security and event management. I lost the first one whilst my wife was pregnant at home with morning sickness. I had developed a porn addiction and was staying back later and later at work to indulge in sinful behaviour.

We have four children but in total, shew was pregnant 6 times. A girl, a boy, then a miscarriage, another girl, another boy then another miscarriage. The more I took on these high-power roles, the less motivation I had to be a husband and a father. I began to feel lost, trapped in a world with no way out as divorce, for me, was not an option.

I searched for identity in my career, putting on a show and pretending to be happy as a family man. I was never able to feel or express love though. My lustful feelings towards other females grew and the predatory instincts I had developed were escalating.

After several flirtatious engagements with females at work, church, and through social media, I commenced an affair with a female who was not only the wife of a friend, but who was also a friend of my wife. Inevitably, the relationship between my wife and my affair partner dwindled. My wife questioned the reason for the breakdown in their friendship but had no idea of the truth.

I was not meeting my wife's emotional needs and was frustrated at not being happy, taking my frustrations out at home by being snappy, demanding and controlling. The affair partners started to grow, as did my inappropriate behaviour at work. Only one of the six affair partners I had was a one-night stand, but it was premeditated. The others were medium-term relationships but with no real sense of emotional attachment or love from my end.

My third affair partner became pregnant and miscarried. My wife found out about this and confronted me after she had been prompted by God to check my phone one night, in addition to my mood swings and secretive behaviour increasing. I confessed to the affair but lied about the fact that there had been others. I even manipulated the counsellor we were seeing to place more blame on my wife than on me. My wife forgave me, and we stayed together with our four children.

For a while, our relationship seemed to improve. I did not stop my adulterous behaviour though, and just became better at hiding what I was doing and manipulating the situation. The affairs would validate me making me feel better about myself for a short period of time. I was in control. They would do what I wanted, when I wanted it. They became a place of escape which I would run to more often. There was still unbelievable amounts of guilt and shame and I would beat myself up on the inside, then after the bad feelings subsided, I'd repeat the cycle all over again.

Living a lie in a house with a Christian family, I constantly felt bad, feeling that when you are bad, God doesn't want to know you. I knew I had to stop and seek God's forgiveness, but I hid from Him because I feared His response to me.

I fought to portray an image where I did not look so bad, going through life trying so hard to manage expectations and manage behaviours so I can look okay.

I was trapped by my fear. To allow God in my life meant giving up control and this terrified me.

My sixth and final affair partner also became pregnant and went through with an abortion. Her husband, also a friend of mine, found out about the affair and alerted my wife. I initially tried to lie and manipulate the story but was resigned to the fact that my wife was not going to be fooled by any more lies. I had already had my second chance and was sick of living a lie with a black cloud always heavy on me.

I sat down with my wife and confessed every sexual sin that I had conducted through our relationship (as much as I could remember). I moved into the spare room, and we lived together for a year separately for the sake of co-parenting our children. We undertook counselling separately. I left my position at work and took on a new role with less power and responsibility.

Despite my efforts trying to change, I actually wasn't and at home, I was showing no remorse and was not changing who I was on the inside. I became part of a Men's Group in September 2019 and my wife moved out of the family home with the children. I was advised that the marriage was over and that we would just co-parent.

Come December 2019, I resorted back to my selfish desires and started a relationship which I kept hidden from everyone. I knew it was wrong and would not help in getting my family back. I did it anyway as I was lonely and still not willing to submit to Christ.

When my wife asked, I told her about the relationship and from that point forward, I could tell that my wife had 0% interest in a romantic relationship with me or sharing anything about herself with me. I was disgusting to her.

Shalom House had been planted in my mind over several years by many people and I had been following Shalom on Facebook for a while. On the day, I completed a medical examination for a new FIFO job that I was starting, I saw a Facebook post advertising the Men's 'Get A Life' camp in Busselton starting the following day. I called Pete and was given directions to turn up at his place the following morning, which I did.

I arrived at camp and was blown away by the atmosphere, despite having judged Shalom as something that was not for me, because I was not a substance abuser or convict. I felt like this was a place where I belonged.

The openness, honesty and integrity of every man at the camp was something that I have never experienced before and allowed me to open up and see that I am not alone in my struggles. I resonated with several of the testimonies that were shared on camp and made connections with fellas whom I still talk to today. I had some powerful group and one-on-one chats and came to an understanding that sin is sin. My sin is no worse or better than anyone else's. I had a couple of big revelations occur and was left feeling like, "I can't keep doing the things that I was doing, I need Shalom!"

On Monday morning as we were packing up to return to Perth, I expressed my desire for help and was accepted into the program, handing over my keys and phone. My intake date was 30th of November 2020 and since then I have had a lot more revelations through the Word and from gaining a better understanding of my past condition.

Early on, I found the program easy to submit to as I was not buckled and found comfort in the regimented routine, having had a security background.

I was coherent, understanding, committed to doing one day at a time to get through and restore the mess I had made. I worked, and I am still working on my relationship with God/Jesus, which I have never had before.

On my first Home Leave, four months in, I spent a weekend with my family celebrating one of my children's birthdays. This was the first time walking back into the family house and the first time my eyes were really opened to the destruction my actions had caused. I felt out of place (in my own home) and really unsure in my role and knew that I had a long way to go.

Shalom enabled me to maintain contact with my children and through the early stages, thanks to their Mum for bringing them. I was able to spend time with them on Saturdays at family church and speak to them on the phone during the week. I was able to sit in front of the mother of my children and finally take full responsibility for my actions, showing remorse for what I had done and then on a separate occasion, hear how my actions had affected my wife and how they made her feel.

As I progressed through Stages 2 and 3 of the program, I went out to paid work, from 2 days a week, to 3 and then 4, but was quickly starting to feel that I could be getting more out of the program if I was still around the operations.

When I hit Stage 4 in October 2021, I commenced as a Truck Leader with Shalom Works and took on the Head Truck Leader position shortly after. I was able to see my children every weekend on my rostered days off and upon reaching Stage 5, I have assisted them with their home schooling on Monday afternoons.

I reached Stage 5, 13 months into the program, at Christmas 2021 and currently still serve as the Head Truck Leader, leading a team of 7 trucks, discipling Truck Leaders and men at lower stages of the program and being the go-between for the trucks with other departments/office. I lead the Shalom sports teams and still do regular mentoring as there are challenges faced every week.

At Christmas 2021, I was able to do reconciliation with my siblings, who I had judged based on their faith values not aligning with mine, thus feeling they could not assist me, and who I had not been there for emotionally or in person when required. I have since worked on my communication with my siblings and regularly catch up with them now for dinner and/or games nights. At the 16-month mark, I lost hope of a reconciliation of my marriage, believing that my desire to want to fix what I had broken was selfish in a way, thinking that if it was all made right again, that I would be okay and would not be judged as a failure. I am committed 100% to being the best parent I can be and working with my ex-partner to raise our children in the best way possible.

I have recently moved out of the Men's housing to a 4x2 house in Aveley which I share with another Stage 5 and I am excited about this new chapter in my life. I start Bible College in Semester 2 and am enjoying coaching junior sport again on Saturday mornings (my daughter's soccer team). Through Shalom, I have been able to humble myself, trust others and trust God, giving up all the control I had over my own life. I now experience emotion and have surrendered everything to God to control. I am in a place where I can feel love and I am working on being able to express love to my brothers in Christ. I was baptised on Christmas Day in 2020 along with my eldest daughter and know that in Jesus, I have all that I need.

I still have relationships to restore but trust the program. I am taking one day at a time and learning not to look at the old me, tainted with sin, but to live and walk in the light, living righteously and with joy.

Shalom House is 'Leading the way in Holistic Rehabilitation.'

BRANDON'S STORY

Hi, my name is Brandon. I am 23 years of age and before I came to Shalom House, I was completely lost, I'd burned every bridge, my relationships were toxic. I was a liar, everyday weed smoker, I manipulated doctors to get meds such as dexies and Ritalin, and while I wait for the next batch, I relied on the streets for methamphetamine.

My problem was just about everything, drugs, sex, rock 'n' roll, and ANGER...I hated the world and I hated myself. I had done a lot of things that made me feel a lot of shame. Growing up, I treated people the way I was treated, playing mums and dads, crossing the boundaries of kids and being surrounded by people who were like-minded.

I moved to Australia from South Africa at the age of 10 and I was raised in Armadale (say no more). So, before Shalom, I had an ongoing drug and anger problem for about seven years. I couldn't finish what I started ever, whether that be a relationship, job, anything. I had been an apprentice plumber for seven years because drugs always got in the way of me holding down a job. I even lost my dream car.

So just before Shalom, I was at the bottom of the bottom, I had no one, my house was completely trashed. I was running from the shadow people and people who didn't exist were out to get me, in a deep psychosis. So, I called PLJ. Shalom shaved my head and gave me a bed (goodbye mullet). This is my second attempt at the program and I'm nine months in, but since the start, I've been a part of Shalom House for almost two years. Since then, I have come a very, very long way.

My life has changed drastically. First and foremost, I found God! I have an everlasting relationship with Jesus, my Lord and Saviour. The power of the life-giving spirit has set me free from the power of sin that leads to death (Romans 8:2).

Thanks to Shalom, I have my life back, I've been reconciled with my family and our trust has been restored. I've been blessed with a car and my plumbing apprenticeship is back on track and when I look at my contact list, I feel so blessed. I am surrounded by love. I have overcome anger, most of it anyway,   and   I'm   just happy to be back.

Shalom House is 'Leading the way in Holistic Rehabilitation.'

TESTIMONY OF TERESA

My name is Teresa, I am 54 years old. I am a part of the Ladies Program here at Shalom House. I grew up in Perth, West Australia, youngest of four girls to Polish parents. My Mother and Father worked hard for a better life here in Australia, my mother had a very busy traditional life, at home, work and her family in Poland. Hence being extremely busy with a very bad temper, I was very frightened of her, which caused me to become anxious. I was also sexually abused by one of my father's friends for many years.

I have two beautiful adult children, 29 and 31, a boy and a girl who rang Shalom due to me having an initial addiction for 38 years to prescription medication. For the five years before coming to Shalom, alcohol and meth were my addictions until last year in July. If my sister had not rung and I did not answer her phone call, I would have been dead now, even though my two grandchildren are my everything. I was very unhappy with myself for having such a long addiction.

I am very blessed that I have a big family and friend network who love and support me here in Shalom House, my children visit nearly weekly, and I have one weekend a month home visit with my son or daughter which is beautiful. They know how sorry I am that I let them down time and time again, they do say how much I loved them though.

Being in Shalom has brought me closer to God, He has saved my life. I always knew Jesus and cried out often to my God, please help me. Shalom House has helped me in so many ways to unpack all my childhood traumas, thanks to God and my Mentor. I got to forgive my mother and the abuser from my childhood. Shalom House has also given me the tools to cope with my anxiety and just to be calm and slow down. I love reading the Bible, Holy Spirit gives me wisdom.

Shalom House and Jesus have saved my life and the lives of my beautiful family. Thank you for listening.

Bless you all. Amen.

TESTIMONY OF RICKI-LEE

Hello, my name is Ricki-lee. I'm 28 years old, single with no kids. I had a really good upbringing, unfortunately Mum and Dad broke up when I was very young but Mum met another beautiful man that I look up to as a strong father figure. Grew up in Dwellingup, went to a Catholic school. No real issues growing up. Found marijuana at around 17 and soon enough, methamphetamine.

Before coming into Shalom, I was at the bottom of the bottom. Almost every door had been shut to me. I bounced from family member to family member, including my sisters. That was my last resort. I called Mum and said I wanted to change and I meant it this time. She told me I had to ring Shalom, so on the 31st of August 2021, I was finally accepted into the Shalom program.

Coming into Shalom is one of the hardest things I have ever done, but I sucked it up and realised that this was my consequence for 10+ years of abusing not only drugs but dragging my family behind me. Shalom has helped me to see things that I couldn't see, mentoring has played a major part in my recovery. From day one, I have opened my heart, not only to GOD but to my mentors. Things that I have never talked about have been put on the table and it is honestly freeing.

As my journey in Shalom moves forwards I became extremely hungry for the Word, reading it day and night, knowing that the only way I was going to survive my newfound life was to build a solid foundation. It starts with the Word. I find myself meditating on Matthew 7:29, the wise in the foolish builders: "...storms of many sizes may come but if your foundation is solid nothing will shake you."

I have grabbed onto every opportunity that Shalom offers, I have found myself in leadership. Leading leaders, discipling the people behind me while being discipled by the people in front of me.

I have done Bible College for more of an insight into the Word. I found myself at paid work with the opportunity to start an apprenticeship but at the end of the day, I didn't come into Shalom to make money. I came to change my life. So back I came into the protective bubble of Shalom. I've really opened up to Jesus as my LORD and Saviour. I'm not only a Leader in the House, but a leader in the church as well. I'm slowly sorting out my debt but that will come with time, not my time but the LORD'S time. My inner spirit is hungry and as strong as ever, knowing that to keep my cup topped up, I have to feed that spirit.

Keeping my eyes on Jesus as I go about my day, Shalom is not only changing my life, but is changing my family's life as well. My Mum doesn't stress about me every night, no longer thinking that there's gonna be a knock on the door late at night to be told I'm dead and that serious stuff because it's so true. She knows I'm safe and that she's getting her boy back, Slowly but surely, she's seeing changes. If I would have any motivational words for people out there struggling with life-controlling issues, it would be: "You can change."

If I can change and come from the bottom of the bottom, then anyone can.

It's okay not to be okay and there's people out there that really do care about you and want the best for you. I've learned that you have to love yourself before you can love anyone else, I've learned to speak words of affirmation over myself on a daily basis, motivation myself with uplifting words.

I'm super grateful for Shalom, for Peter and Amanda, all the volunteers and everyone else that makes Shalom run. Shalom has such a unique culture and if you let the program do what the program is meant to do, it will change you.

Thank you from the bottom of my heart.

GEORGE'S TESTIMONY

Hello, my name is George, my journey at Shalom started around six years ago and this is my second attempt at getting my life together. Six years ago, I was stuck in a dark place consumed by thoughts of suicide and stuck in the heavy addiction of alcohol and weed all the time just running from myself.

I've made just about every mistake known to man, I've Hurt people, I've robbed people, people have even died because of my choices. Anyway, I don't want to go too much into my past, you can pretty much picture the type of person I was and the life that I led.

I first came to Shalom in 2015. Honestly, I wanted to change my life, but I still had some serious criminal charges that I was facing and I was also trying to avoid going to prison again. I've spent 13 years of my adult life inside, so was I in Shalom for all the right reasons? At first, I don't believe so and I spent many days thinking that prison was an easier option than being around all those wackos. But as time went on, my thinking became a lot clearer, good things were happening in my life and I felt I was building a relationship with God. I had been in the program for two years, stuffing my pockets and essentially just ticking boxes trying to impress PLJ with how well I could run a House, how well I could organise and run events. "Look at me, look at me!!"

Yeah, I could do all these things really well, but I was still rotten inside, rotten to the core. I hadn't dealt with any of my issues such as judgement, taking offence, forgiving myself, my heart was still a mess. Then a few things started happening around Shalom that didn't concern me. I didn't even know the full details and I started doing a lot of assuming which brought up a lot of judgement, bitterness, anger and resentment which I didn't know how to deal with correctly. So with a gut full of offence and judgement in me, I took off from Shalom. And with all that resentment, bitterness and judgement in me, I was straight back on the drugs and alcohol, the safe, comfortable place, the place I knew.

This continued for three years, it got to the point where I had no concern for my own safety, let alone others. I was reckless, out of control, pushing everyone away to the point where there was only one person in my life that actually cared about me. But I was that caught up on my path of self-destruction that I pushed her away as well to the point where she moved to Melbourne where she is stuck until this day due to Covid.[1]

I've always been very high functioning. High functioning on the outside, holding down a job, renting my own house, on top of all my bills, but I still had this big hole inside of me. It didn't matter how much gear, alcohol or weed that I would pour into my system, I still had this insatiable thirst that could never be quenched and I

---

[1] Written during pandemic restrictions covering interstate travel.

was at the end of myself. So one day when I was at work, I made a pact with myself if I went home to the empty house that day, I was gonna end it.

But I just had this little voice in the back of my head, it just wouldn't go away, "Drop your pride, drop your pride, you are not that important."

It just wouldn't go away. I didn't want to kill myself so the only other option was to drop my pride, apologise to Peter and ask for his help. I did that reluctantly with tears and snot running out of my head. I made the call that I know saved my life.

So I got off the phone to Peter, turned around and my boss was right there and I just told him that I was sorry but I was leaving. This was at 9:30 in the morning. So I went home, put a few things in my bag and headed out to the valley. I've been back for six months now and it's only the last few weeks when I really feel like I'm getting what this program is about. That's only come to my realisation as I've been honest with my Mentor about my life-controlling issues, and issues that are coming up for me as I'm on this journey this time, such as abandonment, an issue that I didn't even realise was there.

Offence, it's been there all my life. People have been offending me and I'll just put them in the blonk box, put a wall up, problem solved. Now I feel I've got my inner peace back, the more right choices I keep making. God is revealing himself even more and more to me and it's just awesome as a human. Pride is something I have to deal with daily and I just asked God every morning to show me more humility, Lord and the more he does, the more I see the beauty in others for once in my life. I wake up now. Not fearful because I'm in the clutches of addiction or I'm not fearing who I'm gonna hurt today just so I can fulfil my selfish desires.

And I feel I can be a positive influence on others just by the way I live my life now.

The last thing I want to say is "Thank you, God, thank you for taking my weakness, my brokenness and turning it around for good and thank you for revealing yourself to me every day.

Thank you for walking with me every day and being a part of everything I do.

JOSHUA'S STORY

G'day, my name is Joshua, born May 2002 in a small town an hour south of Perth called Rockingham. I grew up in a family of four.

I started my schooling at Safety Bay Primary School where I developed most of my sporting skills along with my Dad teaching me every day after school (Aussie Rules), I have played football from a very young age up until the age of 17 for two local clubs, Safety Bay Stingers and Rockingham Rams.

I studied high school at Rockingham Senior High School where I was involved in a Marine program in Year 8, then joined the Basketball program in year 9. I also played basketball from a young age but didn't take it as serious as Aussie Rules until Year 9 at school where I would train twice every day and have games twice a week. I played two years in a row in the state championships in Melbourne under the Australian Institute of Sport, with some of the best memories of my life being on these trips.

I have always loved fishing, going out on Dad's boat from a young age, mainly catching King George Whiting and Herring. My parents split up when I was 10 which made everything more difficult for me and my sister.

In the late years of high school, I tried a little weed, my use grew and grew along with alcohol. I kept switching between the two and

I would try to give up the weed then keep relapsing, going through this cycle since Year 11 up until the day I came into Shalom. From January 2021, I worked FIFO as a Traffic Controller earning a decent wage which I blew on drugs and alcohol. I quit my job in November 2021 and became more addicted to the weed, living off my Mum's money after I blew all my work money, using her car when mine wouldn't work. Everything just went really bad, and it was all happening in my Mum's house.

Then I hit the brick wall. Mum wouldn't give me any more money and no one wanted me in their house under the influence because I just kept asking for money everywhere I went, house to house. So, me, my Mum, my sister, and Dad decided to look into rehabs. My Dad had heard of Shalom on a few radio stations, so the next day after hearing about Shalom, I called up and spoke to Peter Hempsell and spilled out my problems then put me straight through to PLJ and he asked me to come straight up to the office that day. It was the ninth of April at lunchtime and I had an interview which, little did I know, was going to be my intake straight after.

I got my hair chopped off. For months, my mum was asking me to get a haircut prior to me coming into Shalom. I also got my phone confiscated which I am so thankful for because I was addicted to it.

Shalom has helped me in so many ways. I am honestly speechless about my experiences so far. For starters, I am substance-free in a secure, and safe drug-free environment with the biggest support base anyone could ever wish for. I am a productive member of society, not sitting in a shed anymore.

I have a bed to sleep in at night, food for breakfast, lunch and dinner, showers, clothes if needed, honestly, all you could wish for and paying only $300 a week. My personality has changed so much, I have gained a huge connection with God. I am a Christian, when before meeting God, I would never have thought to become a Christian. I am so, so thankful He has taken me on this journey to Shalom because it has honestly changed me in my flesh and in my spirit hugely. I have gained massive faith in Jesus Christ, and I am so blessed to be a part of the Shalom bubble.

I would like to express to anyone struggling in any way that Shalom has changed my life in such a short period. It's so worth every second, every dollar. From my experience so far, if you open your heart and receive from God through the bible or prayer, I guarantee you at some point in your walk/ journey you will be restored through the mind, flesh and spirit (Romans:12:2,8).

Shalom House is 'Leading the way in Holistic Rehabilitation.'

ALYCE'S STORY

Hi, my name is Alyce. I am 28 years of age, will be 29 in December. I was in addiction for 14 years starting with weed, ending in the heaviest of heavy drugs being heroin, Xanax, meth, you name it in the end. A bottle of Xanax was my go-to daily, all the possible meth and smack too. Before coming to Shalom, I was the biggest trainwreck mess, I was at the bottom of the bottom, I was in a bad relationship, was violent and involved in a lot of crime and drugs.

When I came into Shalom, I was barely functionable. I was in and out of hospital having bad seizures. I would drop to the floor in the blink of an eye. I vomited for the first six weeks, day in, day out. I honestly thought my detox was going to kill me, it was the hardest thing I have ever experienced. I have three children, 10, 6 and 5. I hadn't seen my 5- and 6-year-olds for almost two years, but since coming to Shalom, I have had that restored and will be getting them back in two months' time. I have just gotten my eldest son back full time.

I have been in Shalom House for eight months now and have received and achieved more in this short time than I ever have before in my life. Shalom House is the best thing I have ever done, it has saved my life, restored my family and much more. I have also gained a great relationship with God and that is only getting stronger every day. Without Him I would be dead, not only has Shalom House impacted me but it has impacted my family, also my kids have a massive curiosity in God and want to know Him more and more. My Mum and Dad have also opened their hearts more to God.

The change in me is amazing, I am one of many who are living proof that this program works — you must stick it out and go through the fire, not around it or avoid it. To deal with your life issues and the spots on your heart is hard, but so rewarding. I pray on a daily basis that our Lord makes a way for all the people in addiction at the bottom of the bottom, also for their family members too.

Thanks for reading and God Bless. Alyce.

Shalom House is 'Leading the way in Holistic Rehabilitation.'

EMMA'S STORY

Before entering Shalom on 02/08/21, I was living in a small 2-bedroom unit sharing with two other guys — one who was my brand-new drug dealer who I'd just met. I was sharing my room and a single bed with my teenage son who was also homeless. Life was a complete mess. For the past six months, I'd been floating from place to place since I'd left Shalom in February 2021.

I'm Emma, this is 7th (and final) attempt at rehab. I'll be 35 at the end of the year, I've been at Shalom House for almost a year. My 12-year-old daughter came to live with me here at Shalom after I'd been here for three months. It was unexpected — but such a Godsend and honestly, a pivotal part in helping me to stick it out here at Shalom.

I was introduced to meth when I was 27 and after my marriage of 10 years had completely broken down. After using substances like dexamphetamines and marijuana since my early teens, I justified 'experimenting' with meth at 27, but it quickly became my obsession and after a year, I was injecting it.

I am in shock as I sit here and add up all the years — 8 years — that have been wasted living in this hell. My two children were taken from me numerous times in this period and they were shifted from family member and back again, while I was absent from their lives. Can I just say how grateful I am to every family member who helped or was involved in some way with my kids — thank you and I'm sorry.

I was pretty broken after my marriage failed. Our relationship was toxic, violent, abusive and controlling. I had some pretty deep-seated darkness and lies I believed about myself. The low self-esteem and self-hate, shame and guilt I carried around kept me in the cycle of self-destruction. The times where I didn't have kids in my care also led me deeper into using and hanging around unsavoury people.

I started using heroin for a short period and at the time, I didn't care if I overdosed. Thankfully, I stopped that, but my meth habit increased and I became so miserable and also quite psychotic. I was also contemplating prostituting myself after already doing it a couple of times in exchange for drugs. The fact that I was doing this was a red flag that I'd dropped to the bottom of the bottom.

My character was completely compromised and I was turning into someone I hated. My teenage son was also going down a similar path of addiction and getting in trouble with the police. It was after talking with him that I decided to go back to rehab and finish what I started.

Shalom has helped me to find me. The encouragement that you are surrounded with daily by a community of total support, you can't quite find anything like it. The comforting routine of cleaning, cooking, working, church, it all helps build my confidence that I can actually function and be a productive, helpful and useful person without using drugs.

I am so thankful to be able to do something that I love and am passionate about. Being 2ic at the café has helped me massively with my self-confidence. I thoroughly enjoy my job and feel privileged to be able to make the cakes and I show some flair.

I love that my daughter has embraced the Shalom program and we get to be a family again. I love taking and picking her up from school, she got an outstanding report card from her 1st Semester in high school. I took her to the movies on the weekend. I love that I have the money to do things like that with my daughter and not have to be high to do it. I can pay for her school uniforms and school fee, something I couldn't manage before.

I was blessed with a car early in the year, it's been a massive part in me re-building my new life, being able to take my daughter out and using my car for good things and not a vehicle to pick up and chase drugs around is a huge thing. I visited my Mum a couple of weeks ago and pulled into her driveway and when she greeted me like, "Hello my responsible daughter," it touched my heart. In all my brokenness, I always tried to put up an appearance and make it look like I was somewhat responsible.

I've had a phone and car now for some time and I know I've changed and am changing because I am careful about the responsibility I've been given. I'm careful with what I watch, what I listen to, how I speak and how I think.

I am also learning to communicate in a healthier way, bringing the truth in love like Jesus would. I've been a massive people-pleaser in the past, letting people trample all over me. Now that my self-esteem is improving, I'm able to set healthier boundaries.

So, I'm very new on this journey of re-building my life, but I just put one foot in front of the other and take one day at a time.

Putting all my trust in God and thankful for His grace, that's what's carrying me through. I know He's got good plans for me and my children, better than anything I've ever done so I'll just keep following Him, He knows what He's doing.

Shalom House is 'Leading the way in Holistic Rehabilitation.'

LYALL'S STORY

My name is Lyall. Just before coming into Shalom, I was in Kalgoorlie, living and working, I was in a very dark place, heavily addicted to drugs, namely methamphetamine. I knew I was about to lose my job because I was having too much time off work and my employer made me get help. My circle of good friends told me to get help and go to rehab.

Shalom has helped me change my life by helping me deal with issues that were causing me to use drugs, such as the death of close relatives, fear of rejection and abandonment. I didn't grow up with Mum and Dad, running away at the age of 16 years old. At Shalom, I have learned to love myself and my confidence has grown. I feel that I am a part of a larger family here.

My relationship with my Mum is back on track and we are talking again. She has peace in knowing I am not doing drugs anymore. I am now debt free for the first time in over 15 years. This is a real weight lifted off my shoulders. I have a solid relationship with God. I pray and read my Bible every day, where I believe having God in my life has given me the strength to overcome my addiction and daily challenges that arise.

I feel very excited for my future as I am about to start full-time study in mental health. I want to be able to help make a change in the Aboriginal community as I see there is a huge need.

I would like to tell others that it is never too late to make a change in your life. No matter what you have done or where you have come from, there is an army of people equipped and willing to help you at Shalom House.

Shalom House is 'Leading the way in Holistic Rehabilitation.'

TINA'S STORY

My name is Tina Cole, I'm 50 years old and I am the oldest of 3. I grew up in a lot of dysfunction from childhood to adulthood. Growing up, I was made to feel like I didn't matter and most of the time, I was brushed off by those who were supposed to care and love me, so I grew up angry and hating on everyone. All I know is that I was hurting, broken, and abused. This is just a little bit about me and where I came from and how it affected my direction in life.

Before coming to Shalom, I was living between my Mum's and my brothers, before that I was in Gosnells in a (Homes West) department housing unit where I only stayed for four months due to drugs and alcohol. I got myself into a lot of trouble and had to move out.

My brother told me about Shalom House and the Ladies Program. For a few months, my brother kept sending me the link and photos of the ladies in Shalom, it drove me nuts. I hit rock bottom at my brother's place and he kicked me out when we had a fight. I was seeing and hearing things and was extremely paranoid at this stage.

I walked around for the night, it was cold and raining and I just started crying. I was just so tired and exhausted. I knew I had to go back to my brother's place and beg for him to let me stay the night and I knew I had to get help, so my brother took me in that night. The next morning, I made the call. Next thing I know I was at Shalom having a so-called interview. LOL, yeah nah, it's not how I thought it would go, but I'm glad at the time I didn't know what was going on.

The first few months of being in Shalom House was really hard for me. I had to learn the culture and it took a bit of getting used to, I had such a battle in my head to stay or go, I knew I was fighting for my life eventually. Bit by bit, I started to accept that this was where I needed to be, not just for me but to also heal my family. I didn't want to lose them. I had done so much damage and made their lives miserable and unbearable.

I have my family back in my life, they cannot believe how much I have changed. They now trust me in their homes, giving me the house keys. I never thought that would happen, my family are so proud of me and are so happy. But most of all, my family is fully restored and happy they don't have to worry about me anymore.

Being at Shalom, I stopped a lot of my swearing and angry outbursts and gained a new way of thinking. I realised my anger was because I was a scared child inside who had never healed, although being in Shalom, I have also learned new tools on how to deal with things that come my way and face them head on.

A lot has changed about me, I'm learning to trust others, my attitude has changed. I'm a lot calmer and happier than I have been for a long time. I'm learning to love myself and like myself more every day.

Every day, I'm healing, getting to the bottom of my pain and in the process, healing my heart. I'm slowly getting my confidence back and feeling and getting stronger every day.

I'm now in Stage 4 in the Ladies Program, I now work in the office as the Program Manager. I'm learning new skills every day in the office. I have now been at Shalom for over a year. I am not the same person who walked into Shalom a year ago. I'm in Leadership at Oasis with some wonderful ladies where I care about all the ladies in the program, they are all amazing and all have a story.

Since being in Shalom, I have completed my Year 10 certificate. I have a lot of support and enjoy being around people who believe in me and have helped me in my journey to turn my life around.

I'm a million miles away from the person I used to be, it's been the hardest thing I have ever had to do for myself, but I know it was God's Plan that brought me to Shalom. He knows what is best for me and I'm listening to what He wants from me and not what I want.

Through what I have learned this past year being at Shalom, I would like to help other ladies to turn their life around, and who better to do that then someone who has.

Thank you for reading my testimony.

Shalom House is 'Leading the way in Holistic Rehabilitation.'

ANDREW'S STORY
Hi, my name is Andrew, I am 41 years old and I'm from Queensland. I have a 23-year-old son is currently residing in Queensland with his girlfriend. Growing up, I had quite a few issues that affected my life, from my parents splitting up, then both my parents having strokes quite young and my youngest brother dying in an accident aged ten.

So our family dynamic got separated and dysfunctional quite quickly. Unfortunately, I didn't cope as well as I actually thought that I did. This led me down a long-winded path of drugs, self-sabotage and eventually, dysfunction.

Before coming into Shalom, I was a full-blown meth addict living out of my car and running around 24 hours a day, selling drugs, committing crimes and scams that either bordered on legal loopholes or were illegal to feed my habit.

Looking back on my old life, I now realise how hard it was to function day to day, trying to make enough money and ends meet to get through to the next day. It was actually quite a stressful full-time job trying to feed my habit. That, coupled with the extreme anxiety and depression from the hopelessness of where my life had ended up, nearly pushed me to suicide many, many times. I used to be a high-functioning drug user who really pushed in to my working life, but a long-term relationship breakup with my son's mother really took a toll on my life and my own self-worth.

That led to a whole series of bad relationships with different girlfriends, different jobs, living in different geographical locations, all the while thinking each time something went wrong, "If I just had (this or this different), I would stop using the drugs."

How wrong I was!!!

Because all the while, not realising that all my problems actually lay within me, I was broken and hurting. I kept trying to run away from everything when things went downhill, looking to change everything but me.

When I first came to Shalom, I was really busted and broken, I felt like I couldn't do anything right. My mind was quite foggy, I couldn't think very clearly and I struggled emotionally and even verbally to communicate.

I have paid off about half of my $50,000 debt in the last 20 months since coming to Shalom. Relationally with my family, things have never been better. I had a Home Leave back to Queensland in May 2022. Unfortunately, because of how I use to live, my family were initially apprehensive about me staying for a whole week with them. Yet immediately after the Home Leave, my family asked if I could rebook another Home Leave for Christmas this year for two weeks.

In 2019, I had an encounter with God but I have never had any relationship with him until I entered Shalom. Shalom is a discipleship House. So, reading the Bible and being surrounded by like-minded individuals has strengthened me with a bold faith in Christianity. I am now confident, bold, I have self-worth, and I really love the person that I am becoming. I love how GOD and Shalom are working hand-in-hand in my life to help me to better myself every day.

I want to thank the founders, Pete and Amanda, for all the good works they are doing in my life and the lives of others. I encourage anyone who has a life-controlling issue out there who doesn't know where to go and get help that Shalom will help you. It is a very hard and tough program, but by coming to Shalom you have nothing to lose and yet everything to gain!

Shalom House is 'Leading the way in Holistic Rehabilitation.'

CONGRATULATIONS RYNE

For most people, today is a day to celebrate the end of the week and look forward to resting or celebrating with their loved ones.

For me, today is a special day as it marks two years clean and sober, and as insignificant as this may sound for some, those of you who know me understand this truly is a remarkable achievement. I firstly thank my family for enduring some difficult times, and to everyone else along the way who has had a part of my recovery, you all know who you are 😊 .

I still fall short every day and make mistakes, but I'm very proud of who I've become, and encourage anyone out there struggling with anything to be courageous and speak up. This was my first step to achieving what I have today.

Have a blessed Friday 🩶

Shalom House is 'Leading the way in Holistic Rehabilitation.'

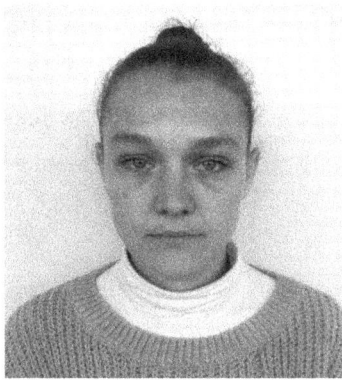

MY NAME IS REBECCA.

I am 29 years old. I was born in a small country town called Moora, but I grew up in Rockingham.

My parents divorced when I was three years old. I was lucky enough to still have my Dad around as my parents always stayed friends for us kids. When I was growing up, my Mum was always depressed, and my dad was a depressed alcoholic. I have an older brother and a younger sister.

I stayed at my Dad's house every second weekend growing up and he joined us on all camping holidays and big family events, Christmas etc. It was nice to still have my Dad around even though it didn't work out with my parents.

One of the weekends at Dad's place, I woke up to someone molesting me. I was frozen still, scared and I didn't know what to do. I don't know how long it took me to tell someone about it, which ended up being hard as it was someone I was really close to.

I don't have many memories, but Mum put me in counselling for it. I just remember hating it. Around the age of ten, I started to get bullied at school. This made me feel so rejected. I felt lonely and not liked, nothing a 10-year-old kid knows how to react to.

When I was 12, I remember my Mum working a lot and she started studying a couple of years later. My Dad never helped financially so she wanted to do the best she could to provide for us kids. This meant I was looking after my little sister a lot, taking her home on buses after school, cooking the dinners. My brother helped a little bit, but I was the main one to do it all. I guess I resented my little sister because I could never hang out with my friends after school and stuff like normal kids would do.

When I was 14, I met my 'First Love'. I ended up being with him for nine years. His family were quite different to what I had been around before. My Mum was quite protective and sheltered me from a lot. His family were all about drugs and could be quite violent towards each other. Little did I know, I was headed down that path. I was shown drugs and was around them a lot from the age of 16.

Weekends were spent going to my boyfriend's house, drinking and having sex with him. A week before my 18th birthday, I decided I was going to smoke my first cone. I liked the feeling of it, so I started doing it socially every weekend.

About the same time, I became the Manager of a Subway store. I loved my job and was very passionate about it. Three years went by and I fell pregnant. I always wanted to be a mum, it's always been at the top of my list. The day I found out the baby had no heartbeat broke me. I'd never felt so heartbroken in my life. We then decided to hit the meth to deal with the pain. Before I knew it, we were selling meth and weed to pay for both our habits. I was a huge pot smoker and pretty big meth user at this stage which led to falling short in my job, stealing from my boss, being violent. My relationship had become so toxic, it was like we hated each other. It was unhealthy and the path we were headed down was scary. I finally had the courage to leave him.

I continued to smoke bongs daily, I was in such a depressed state. I felt like I had nothing: no baby, no job and no man. Out on the town one night, I met who I thought was an amazing, handsome guy. He ended up being a controlling, abusive alcoholic who isolated me from all my family and friends. He made me feel so alone, but at the time I was so broken, and I thought I loved him so much. He made me believe I wouldn't get anything better because I was nothing and no good at anything. My self-esteem and worth were so low. I was so depressed, bitter and angry at the world. We would drink and smoke cones every day, selling pounds of weed driving around all over Perth. To be honest, I don't know how I didn't kill myself or someone else driving while so intoxicated. Thinking back, it makes me sick.

The cops were called out for domestic violence all the time by our neighbours. I then fell pregnant to him, and he forced me to get an abortion, knowing I had miscarried in the past. I somehow allowed this to happen. I hated myself for this and lived with that guilt every day, which meant the weed use became heavier to mask even more of my pain. I then finally found the courage to get away from him. Deep down, I still 'loved' him and cared for him, which I hated myself even more for, so I promised myself I would never fall in love again.

I then started sleeping around, with one of the men being a friend of my boyfriend's, which is something I would never normally do. I continued to drink and smoke weed every day, then picked up the meth every now and then. I was on the road to self-destruction. I was numb and didn't care about anything or anyone. I then met this other guy and we had good times in the bedroom, so I kept seeing him. Before I knew it, I was using meth daily.

He used to lock me in rooms, beat me until I was hospitalised, took my phone away from me. It turned out even worse. I just kept ending up in these toxic situations because I was on such a dark path and hated myself. Inside, I was hoping he would kill me. I attempted suicide three times in six years whilst being on this self-sabotaging path.

My family had turned their backs on me as they couldn't stand to see me on such a self-destructive path and they just didn't know what else to do any more. I felt so alone and worthless, it was horrible. I ended up witnessing a very traumatic event which led to this guy becoming comatose. I had hit rock bottom. After this I was completely fried, seeing things that weren't there and hearing voices.

I called my Mum and begged her for help. Thank God she accepted. She took me to Rockingham Hospital because of the state I was in. I ended up in the mental ward. My Aunty then told me about Shalom. I had two other Rehabs taking me in at this stage, but something in my head was telling me I had to go to Shalom. For the first week, I thought, "Where have I put myself? These people are crazy thinking God's just going to fix all their problems." I was still respectful towards everyone and did the daily devos that were required. It felt like I was reading a different language, I couldn't really connect to any of it. On Thursday night, we went to Brittany's House for group. I had no idea what this was going to be like.

We ate some food, had a chat and then they put the worship music on. I didn't know what came over me. I was bawling like a baby the whole way through to these songs that I didn't even know. So, after that Brittany and Nicola asked me if they could pray for me and I said they could straight away. So they prayed, and I can't explain the feeling that I got inside, I was so hot and sweaty and I had like hot tingling feelings across my upper back. It was an amazing feeling. I was so overwhelmed by the supernatural feeling I got by what I know and couldn't deny was the Holy Spirit.

A week went on and that next Thursday morning, I packed my bags and was adamant that I was going home. I couldn't comprehend the love God gives us and the freedom of shame and guilt He offers us. I got scared and was about to run like I would have in my old life, until Pete asked if I would just spend an hour to hear him out until I made my mind up. In that hour, it happened again. Pete prayed over me, and the same feelings went through my body, and I was an absolute blubbering mess.

Pete spoke about things in my life that he couldn't have known. I hadn't told anyone at Shalom about them. I was so much lighter and at peace. I know it was God working through him. I know it's God that's allowed me to let go of the shame and guilt I've been carrying onto for years now. I'm so thankful to God and Shalom for allowing me to feel and know the Holy Spirit. I now feel there is a light at the end of the tunnel and I do have purpose in life. I haven't felt as worthless and I love God for all the work He is doing in me. It's only early days and I feel so much calmer and at peace since I've known God.

I am excited and thankful to keep building this relationship with Him. He is amazing and I want to know him more.

I have been in the Shalom Women's Program now for 21 months now and the person I came in as and the person I am today are completely different. I am now free from five addictions. I am free from anger, anxiety and depression. I have built up self-confidence and I can finally say that I am proud of the person I am. I have a sense of peace over me that I have never had before. God has filled that void that I have been trying to fill for nearly my whole life and I now feel like I have a purpose in life.

This journey has been very raw, emotional and challenging but they have been the best times of my life and I am genuinely happy with where my life is now and where it is headed. I have learned so much since being in Shalom, communicating is one of the biggest. I am now one of the Leaders in the Women's Program and I am honoured to be able to help those coming behind me.

My family relationships that I thought were ruined forever are being restored, friendships from school and those from when I was a child are being restored, I have a full-time position at the Shalom Café, I have been blessed with a car, my debt that I thought I would never be able to catch up with is getting paid off and I have only people around me who truly care about me.

God is doing so much in my life, and I am so thankful to have met Him, I love Him and all glory to Him, I could not have done all of this in my own strength. I finally feel like I fit and I am not just a burden to people. I am not sure what God has planned for my future, but I am confident that it's good and I'm excited about the journey to get there. Thank you to Pete and Amanda and everyone that has been part of my journey so far. I couldn't have done it without you all.

DEE'S TESTIMONY

I was born in Bunbury in the mid-70s. My parents said I was a planned baby, I always say not everything goes as planned. My Mum had a troubled birth with me. When I was born, I was not breathing for a long time and they told my Mum that I was probably going to have learning difficulties. It didn't help when I almost drowned in the family pool when I was about three years old. My Mum revived me, she was a lifesaver but I had been without oxygen for a very long time.

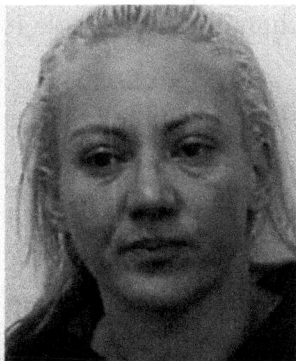

My parents separated when I was very young. My dad was a heavy drinker. He always said he didn't want kids. My Mum and Dad used to fight often. My earliest childhood memories are being sexually abused by a family member when I was very young. Also waiting outside the pub, in the car with my Mum who was always angry with my Dad. My Dad almost running my Mum over when she was walking up one of the main roads in Bunbury one night. I also remember the many beltings I got as a kid.

The same year my parents separated, I was diagnosed with dyslexia. I wondered why I was different from other kids. I was always separated from the other kids at school, always sitting at the front of the class, facing the wall. I was THAT KID the other parents didn't want their kids to play with. I used to hear other parents say things like, "She's not a bad kid, she's just misunderstood."

My school reports always came home with, "She needs to try harder," written on them. I used to think, "I've tried the hardest I can, I'm stupid and will always be stupid."

So, from a really young age, I always felt really different from the other kids, always thought I was stupid. I felt ugly. Why was I so different from the other children?

I remember laying in my bed at night and I would always wonder why I was so different, why wasn't I lovable? I just wanted to die. Before I even started on my drug path, I was plagued with suicidal thoughts.

My parents acted very toxic towards each other and would speak badly about each other. We would go on access weekends with my Dad and sometimes my Dad would have his guns in the boot of the car when my Mum would open it to get our stuff out. I still remember his gun case.

My Mum eventually remarried, and this introduced another brother and sister into our lives. My step-dad was very strict and the stricter he got, the worse I got. My older brother introduced me to drugs when I was in my early teens. I was already drinking and smoking.

I left home at 15 to live on the streets and I thought life was great at the time: no parents, no restrictions. It wasn't long before I meet my first real boyfriend, we started to use speed and trips. We tried to go up north and get away, but the drugs and friends seems to be the same no matter where we went. We came back to Perth and it wasn't long before I found out I was 13 weeks pregnant. So we were married, had a baby, started using drugs again. Mixed with post-natal depression, my life was spiralling out of control. We separated and I tried again to get away from the drugs, not knowing it was me that was the problem, not the drugs. It wasn't long before I met my second eldest child's Dad. We built a house and things seemed OK, but there was still smoking pot every day and drinking. We separated and I moved towns again ... I'd meet a new man and he would seem to be fun and exciting and all those red flags that you should not date. Well, I ran towards them.

He was fresh out of prison and used drugs every day. He was so violent, I walked on eggshells every day. He confirmed every bad thing I had ever thought about myself: worthless, ugly, useless and even that I should just die. I used drugs every day, nightclub every weekend, raves. Dance music was like a drug to me. I neglected my children, drugs came first. Morphine, pills, speed and then I found meth. We had two more children and I stopped walking on eggshells and started to not care if he killed me. I was in and out of the psych wards. Organised Crime arrested me in 2009 and I remember sitting on my front lawn, thinking if I got out of this alive (as in from my addiction), I will help women in the same situation as me to get out of it. Little did I know a seed was being planted in my heart. I was yelling at the sky as like me 2 clean weeks.

I ended up in prison after being arrested. I had been in there six weeks when the Gideons gave me a Bible. I didn't believe in God, but I took it anyway and I put my name in it and I heard God say to me: "You asked for two clean weeks, and you've had six." I started the Step Up program and learned about God, a forgiving God. I asked God if He could forgive me if I just want to die. But He told me to build. I wasn't sure how to do that. I was born again in prison; however, many people have come across my path to help me rebuild along the way.

I went to rehab in 2010. My Dad became my rock, my biggest supporter, he saw my mess and said he finally found his purpose in life, and it was to help me sort out mine. He bought my kids to see me every weekend. In 2012, I was married again to a graduate from the same program. After we were married, I found out he had never stopped using drugs. The heroin was his first love, it was like being cheated on but with a drug. Our relationship soured and I eventually kicked him out. Three weeks later, he died of a heroin overdose. I was destroyed. I lost my job, my house. I lost myself, but the one thing I held onto was God.

There was a post on Facebook about Shalom wanting to start a female program. I thought I would love to do that, but I had a good job so maybe it was not for me. Someone I knew organised for me to go meet Pete. He offered me a job and said, "You'll get smashed when you come here."

I kind of didn't react, but I knew Pete was right because I knew my life was a mess.

My heart was so broken, I was a broken and angry person. I was wanting so much just to help other women, but I was not ready. God told me if you want to step into what I have for you, you need to be laying down the things that hinder you. I was still angry, drinking, smoking, not respecting myself as a woman. It was a pivotal moment, my life could have gone either way at this point, I had a choice, back to the mud and misery or get some integrity and start walking, put my faith where my mouth was.

In the last four and a bit years at Shalom, I have learned more about myself and my life than in the first 41 years. I've gone from being concerned with the way I look, what people think of me, wanting to have friends, to someone who doesn't have to wear makeup every day, someone who doesn't care if I don't fit the world's idea of beautiful. Most of all, I'm not angry and I don't think about dying every minute of every day.

I've been taught how to communicate with people, how to protect my heart. I've learned that even though I make mistakes, I'm not a terrible, worthless person. The last eight months, we have even been living with a family while our house is being built, we have really learned WHAT FAMILY IS being here.

In 2019, I meet the love of my life. We were friends who went burger hunting together to being best friends who confided in each other, until one day he said we were going to get married. Every day, he reminds me that he loves me. I now know a soulmate builds your soul, not tears it down. I know what unconditional love is. We were baptised together at Christmas 2019 and Pete married us in 2020.

My husband is a God-focused man, also focused on others, a man of his word and also a man of integrity. I've had my three daughters restored to me and three wonderful grandchildren I am Mimi to. I'm really proud of my children and where they are today, despite the life I dragged them through.

Today, I get to do that very seed that was planted in my heart in 2009, I get to speak into ladies' lives, to tell them they are valuable, loved and I get to tell them every day to get up and keep going because the life that God has waiting for them is nothing they have ever experienced before.

It's not about the way you fall, it's about learning why you fell, and how to get up and not fall over the same things again.

I have good real friends who want FOR me, not FROM me. I

have family. I really want to thank everyone who's been pivotal in my journey. My Dad, my children, Jade, Pete and Amanda, Sue VN, Gav and Tam, Carolyn and Dave, and my husband Riz.

My Jesus for seeing me in the darkness and pulling me out.

Shalom House is 'Leading the way in Holistic Rehabilitation.'

CHELSEA'S TESTIMONY (Life-Changing)

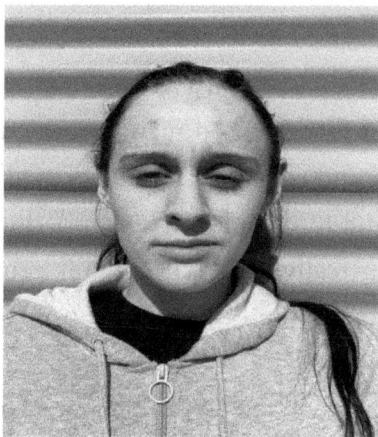

Many people have asked what Chelsea's life was like, well, here is her story, I hope that it encourages you.

Hello, my name is Chelsea, and I am 23 years old, I have three kids, aged 2, 3 and 5. I grew up in Perth and had a good childhood. I always had a roof over my head. Mum and Dad separated before I got to an age where I'd understand and remember things so the idea and knowledge of what a

Dad/Father is and was in a person's life was unknown to me.

My Dad had a very strong personality which didn't match my quiet personality. So being so young and being so scared of family I became very scared of everything and everyone. I was very attached to my Mum and I would scream when others would try and pick me up.

I developed anxiety from a young age which only grew stronger growing up. I struggled with learning things, and I could never process the simplest of things, which gave people opportunities to put me down. I remember from a very young age, hiding under the bed when my Dad was due to collect me and my sister for his weekend with us. Which meant being uncomfortable and scared without my Mum to comfort me and also the entire weekend with my sister being nasty to me without Dad seeing.

My Mum met my step-dad not long after and I remember him being in our home and thinking to myself, "I don't even know his name."

I still had no idea who and what a Dad was and didn't feel comfortable around my own Dad and now there is a man in my life who is (what I could understand at the time) in my Dad's place which made me very angry. The hate and anger I developed for my step-dad began.

With my Mum moving on and meeting my step-dad (which was and is a good thing because she is happy with him and he is an amazing step-dad and husband to my mum), afterwards, her attention towards me shifted. I struggled with separation anxiety as my Mum was my everything and the only thing/place/person that I felt safe and secure and most of all, comfortable.

In Year 6, I started to self-harm. It started out as an accidental paper cut on my forearm. Cutting my arms once a week turned into three times a week and then every day. I found relief in self-harming. I would cover them up for school and at home. I never realised that I had an addiction at such a young age. Being miserable and seeing and expecting the bad in life was what I craved instead of living freely like a normal kid.

At the age of 10, I started drinking alcohol and smoking. I loved the feeling of being drunk and not feeling miserable. That then transferred into me and my friends getting older kids to buy us alcohol and cigarettes which led to us sneaking out and hanging out with older people. I started smoking marijuana at the age of 11. I became a bad alcoholic and stoner very fast, and the weekend drinking and smoking turned into every day. I started going to parties and experimenting with pills and LSD at 13, I was seeking something that would last longer and make my head stop thinking and be blank.

I met a lot of people through my teenage years. I didn't get along with females as such because I grew up around boys. I just wanted to get high or drunk and hang out with mates. I found myself hanging out with boys who did graffiti and who would every now and then use meth. It got to the point where they considered me family, which I was comfortable with. So, I started doing graffiti and earning respect through that. It was during this time I lost a best friend of mine to suicide. This ripped me apart. I wish I could have talked him out of killing himself, or at least tried. I made the decision to use meth, knowing it tears people and their families apart. I didn't care anymore. I developed my biggest and strongest addiction. It caused me to stop drinking, stop smoking marijuana and not try any other drug. I felt like I had finally got the one thing that made me feel all the things that life didn't, which was comfortable and numb.

I met the father of my kids on my 17th birthday. I saw him and fell in love. He had a FIFO job and he was not like the other boys and we had a lot in common. We dated for three months and because he seemed to have it all together, we both decided to start trying for a baby. Little did I know his drug addiction was new, unlike mine. With me not knowing that, I let myself be vulnerable. This led to one day with him blocking me and not talking to me out of nowhere. I remember crying every day and crying myself to sleep because I wanted to be a Mum and knew that it was my purpose to be one.

I knew deep down I was pregnant. I had all the signs and symptoms but being so in denial I kept using and letting myself be treated like I was worth nothing. At 13 weeks, my Mum clicked onto my pregnancy and I then had my date scan booked.

A week before the scan, I met up with the baby's father and told him I was pregnant because that day I had taken a test which came up positive.

His response was, "It's not mine."

That broke me.

Especially because he had no reason to think otherwise. The day of the scan came, and I went to it alone. I got told I was 13 weeks and I saw my little girl and heard her heartbeat which made me so happy and proud. It changed my mindset completely and gave me such joy and strength that I'd be having my daughter, whether or not her Dad was with me.

After my parents processed it all, they didn't think it was right for me to have a baby, as I couldn't even look after myself. I told them that this was what I wanted. I decided I'd be better off leaving and they agreed. I reached out to the Mum of my kid's father and without hesitation, she told me to come over and I could stay as long as I wanted and needed. So I did just that. I got my older sister to take me with my bags packed. I lived there with my kids' father and his family for my entire pregnancy. After having my daughter, her father started abusing me which was a daily thing. It makes me feel sick, knowing for years I stayed with him and had my two sons because I was too scared to leave him. I still battled with my meth addiction which caused me to steal money off my step-dad for years and years.

In November 2020, my step-dad had had enough and told me to leave. As we had agreed ages before, the kids would stay because although I knew they were my kids, they were not my property, and they were safe at Mum's place. My Mum and step-dad knew I had to hit rock bottom before I would get any help, so they kicked me out, which unfortunately caused me to use more. I had nowhere to go but my kid's father's house. I had no one and nothing so I stayed at his house for months. I had never felt so worthless in my life.

One day at his house, my kids came, and they didn't know I was there. Mum didn't know I was there at all until she came to pick them up the next day. My daughter screamed and cried her eyes out, saying, "I just want to hug my mummy and I just want to say goodbye to my mummy."

That was the final straw. I couldn't do it anymore. I walked outside and I told Mum I needed help and I would do anything. She then told me about Shalom House and said she can get me in today and that I just need to make the call. A few days later, I called Shalom and Peter Hempsell put me through to PLJ and he told me to come in the next day. I did and being me, I didn't understand what I agreed to when PLJ asked if I was ready to come in now.

I said" Yes." (Time to change my life)

Shalom is the best decision I have ever made in my life. My relationships with my parents and siblings are restored. I get to see my kids every Saturday and I have never felt so happy and alive before. I can say Shalom House has given my kids back their mother and my family back their daughter. In the nine months since coming into the Shalom House program, I have changed so much. Where I was sick and broken and had forgotten what it was like to have my children in my life, I am now a strong and confident functioning member of society. I don't even feel like I was an addict, I have learned so many life skills in the time have been here. I am now Stage 3 in the program and the first ladies' Truck Leader doing property maintenance. This is a role that has helped me overcome a lot of my lack of self-confidence and my self-doubt. I have received so much love and support in my new role and I am absolutely loving it.

I have also become a Christian since being in the program and have also been baptised, a big part of my journey as a changed person. I have been reconciled with my family and children. My family offered for me to move back home to be with my kids once I reach Stage 5. This is such a privilege as I had lost the trust of my parents a long time ago. I have a life and a future to look forward to. I would like to thank Peter and Amanda for creating a safe place for God to do a work in me and I will forever be grateful. Shalom will always be my family; I can't wait to see what the future holds.

Shalom House is 'Leading the way in Holistic Rehabilitation.'

RICKI'S TESTIMONY

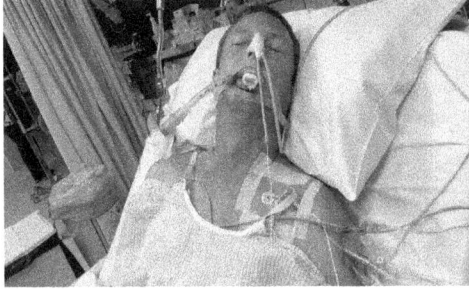

Hi, my name is Ricki Baker and this is my story. My Dad left my Mum before I was born so Mum who was only 18 tried really hard to raise me in the best way she knew how. I was a happy kid who loved playing sports and who was very protective of Mum and kids that were being bullied at school. Back then, I wasn't afraid to stand up and fight back. I was confident and a little bit of a mischief as well, accidentally setting fire to our neighbour's car when I was four.

Growing up, I attended six different primary schools, two different high schools and two schools for troubled kids. I was expelled from three schools for being disruptive and disrespectful. My behaviour started to change around the age of 8 in Melbourne. I was sexually abused by an older girl next door and when we came to Perth, a friend's uncle abused me for a long time. I was too ashamed to tell anyone about what was happening and I started to take it out on Mum and at school.

I managed to make it onto the state basketball team playing for Cockburn Cougars under 13s. I was offered a scholarship, but it was around this time, I was introduced to cigarettes marijuana and alcohol.

I had finally found something that took away the pain of what was happening, my Mum was very strict, and we would often end up having verbal arguments in front of my younger brother and sister. I would get so angry, I would start smashing her stuff until she called the police. I would steal money off her to buy drugs and alcohol and ciggys. Eventually running away for a few months, I finally came back but couldn't live under Mum's strict conditions. We had a massive argument and DCD came and took me to a foster home. I spent two weeks there and then I was taken to a hostel.

In the morning, a guy pulled a knife on me and threatened me for my money. I was alone, scared and getting high and drunk became a daily routine.

I started to get in trouble with the law, stealing cars, doing burglaries and at the age of 14, I progressed to acid and at 15 shooting up amphetamines and occasionally heroin. I would pretty much take anything that would take me away from reality. I had no hope, couldn't hold a job or a girlfriend, my world evolved around drugs. I was selfish and had no regard for my family or the law.

I went to my first rehab at the age of 18, only because Mum was nagging me to go, I didn't really want to stop using. Drugs at that time were fun. I couldn't see the pain I was inflicting on those around me or thinking about how Mum was worried sick at night wondering if she would receive a phone call saying I was in lock up or hospital.

At the age of 23, I went to prison for stealing a car and I didn't really have anywhere to go for parole so I went to Serenity Lodge for a few months. I think that was one of the first times I was clean out in the community and it felt good. I ended up having a few more cracks at rehab but I would never really open up to counsellors about the abuse when I was younger so I was never actually fully healing. Sometimes, I would start to do well for a bit and hold a job for a bit but I would eventually go back to the drugs and lose my job.

Drugs came before rent and I would often find myself getting kicked out. In 2015, Mum was talking about Shalom House. I was kind of interested as I was getting tired of couch surfing and I was seeing my good friends getting married and settling down, having kids and living a normal kind of life. I wanted that as well, it's what I had always wanted but just didn't know how. I knew I needed help and eventually met with Pete.

I didn't realise he wanted me to move in straight away.

I said "Na, I'll come back in two weeks"

He said, "Call me in three months when you are ready."

A couple of months later, I was found dead in the toilet from a heroin overdose. I spent five days in a coma on life support and it took me another 14 months to come back. November 2016, I entered Shalom. I had so much hurt and pain, I was like a broken vase and God was putting me back together piece by piece. For the first time in my life, I was at peace and started to really enjoy hanging out with others- focused people, people who cared and who listened. I was starting to deal with my emotions in a healthy manner and my communication skills were getting better and my time management got better. Me and Mum stopped arguing.

I have learned to trust God as a father who loves me and is not going to leave me and who wants the best for me. He has taught me how to love myself and how to love others. I am currently just over 31 months clean and have my own unit, am attending Bible College and have a full-time job. I get my driver's licence for the first time ever this year and can't wait to see what God has in store for me. Thanks to everyone who has supported me through this journey and who listened, when I was pouring my heart out and crying on to your shoulder. And a special shout out to Pete and Amanda. Words cannot express what this program has done for me and so many families.

Shalom House: 'Restoring the Lives of Men, Women and Children in our Community.'

LIVING WITH A CHILD IN ADDICTION — SARAH

Am I the only one? My heart aches!. My mind races back and forth, in and out. Where did I go so wrong as a mother? Did I fail my child so badly? Did I not do enough? Did I miss something so traumatic in your life?

What went so wrong?

Please, I beg you. just speak to me. Tell me your problems. Let me fix you! Was I the problem all along? Am I still the problem?

All these thoughts. They just don't stop. Lord, make them stop. PLEASE! I beg of you.

It's like a nightmare. I'm on a rollercoaster ride that I cannot get off. Please somebody, anybody...pinch me, wake me from this nightmare.

That rollercoaster ride comes to no end. Not even a second to breathe. Please Lord, breathe your life into me. Because this life is slowly dwindling, going down and I can see no way out.

I try to pretend not to see what's really happening. I try my hardest to believe your manipulative lies...oh, how I want to believe those lies...

That you are okay, that you are still clean.

I look at you and see an empty vessel. Your eyes glazed over with not a hope in sight.

But as I lay in my bed, that bed I cannot get out of. I try to convince myself of the you I once knew...but reality sets in. My own eyes start to glaze over. I'm too, left as an empty shell, seeking something but only emptiness is what I can find. It consumes me. Again, time and time again, I try to break free. When does my own freedom come, Lord? I see no way out.

Alcohol consumes me. My mind is ravaged in only ways you could understand. It's your reality, it is not of my own. Your reality does not even exist. I know this now, but I still can't bring myself to believe what I know to be true. It's far too hard to accept it. My stomach turns at the thought of it.

Because again, am I the cause?

A mother's guilt is sickening. It's gut wrenching to the stomach. It's been so many years, how much more can one take! The devil is having a field day with us. Alcohol and drugs, they are ruining us both. I am the cause. If only I could break the cycle. My child would be FREE...all these thoughts, they just don't stop.

Again, the lies set in. And they hit deep! It drags me down into the pit right next to you. Stop all this madness. I can't take any more, Lord! My way is not working anymore..

PLEASE, have Your way, Your will must be done. Because my ways are not working anymore. This empty vessel is waiting to be filled.

From you, not of this world anymore!

By Sarah Honnor

www.ingramcontent.com/pod-product-compliance
Lightning Source LLC
Chambersburg PA
CBHW072054020426
42334CB00017B/1500